HEAD FIRST

HEAD
FIRST

(HOW THE MIND HEALS THE BODY)

ALASTAIR SANTHOUSE

AVERY
AN IMPRINT OF PENGUIN RANDOM HOUSE
NEW YORK

AVERY

An imprint of Penguin Random House LLC
penguinrandomhouse.com

Most Avery books are available at special quantity discounts for bulk purchase
for sales promotions, premiums, fund-raising, and educational needs.
Special books or book excerpts also can be created to fit specific needs.
For details, write SpecialMarkets@penguinrandomhouse.com.

Library of Congress Cataloging-in-Publication Data

Names: Santhouse, Alastair, author.
Title: Head first: how the mind heals the body / by Alastair Santhouse.
Description: New York: Avery, Penguin Random House LLC, [2021] | Includes index.
Identifiers: LCCN 2020042327 (print) | LCCN 2020042328 (ebook) |
ISBN 9780593188750 (hardcover) | ISBN 9780593188767 (ebook) |
Subjects: LCSH: Mental health services—Evaluation—Great Britain. |
Psychiatry—Great Britain. | Psychiatrists—Great Britain.
Classification: LCC RA790.7.G7 S26 2021 (print) |
LCC RA790.7.G7 (ebook) | DDC 362.20941—dc23
LC record available at https://lccn.loc.gov/2020042327
LC ebook record available at https://lccn.loc.gov/2020042328

Printed in the United States of America
1   3   5   7   9   10   8   6   4   2

Book design by Laura K. Corless

Neither the publisher nor the author is engaged in rendering professional advice
or services to the individual reader. The ideas, procedures, and suggestions contained
in this book are not intended as a substitute for consulting with your physician.
All matters regarding your health require medical supervision. Neither the author
nor the publisher shall be liable or responsible for any loss or damage
allegedly arising from any information or suggestion in this book.

The stories chronicled in this book are based on many years of practice.
However, maintaining patient confidentiality is of utmost importance,
so the author has taken care to remove any identifying clinical or personal information.
Some of the case studies are an amalgam of several patients.

For Sara and the Boys

ASK NOT WHAT DISEASE THE PERSON HAS,
BUT RATHER WHAT PERSON THE DISEASE HAS.

—SIR WILLIAM OSLER, 1849–1919

CONTENTS

CONTENTS

JOURNEY

I remember Roland well, although I met him only twice. In fact, I heard him before I saw him; I was startled by an alarming noise, somewhere between a cough and a snort, as I approached the waiting room on my return from lunch to start an afternoon clinic.

I sat down with him in my consulting room, and he told me his story. Age thirty-three, he was from Gabon, unmarried, and had come to the UK three years earlier. Since his arrival he had experienced increasing discomfort with his throat, resulting in frequent explosive exhalations. His regular doctor had been unable to make a diagnosis and had rather unusually, rather than referring him to a single specialist for an opinion, made three separate referrals.

Roland had found life in the UK difficult. He had struggled to find work, had no family here, and was unable to see his daughter, who lived with an ex-partner in Gabon. His symptoms had begun several years before and were now worse than ever. As he snorted and spluttered, I found myself distracted by a persistent urge to clean my desk with an antiseptic wipe. It was with some difficulty that I listened to his story.

He had been encouraged by friends to see his doctor, who, reading between the lines, hadn't initially worried about his symptoms but had subsequently referred him to the hospital for more opinions.

It was clear to me that the cumulative stress and disappointment in Roland's life had exacerbated a nervous tic, which was now so deeply ingrained in his motor system as to be automatic. I had seen symptoms like this before, in which unusual movements and behaviors, rehearsed often enough, become "hardwired." For example, I have seen people present with a strange gait that makes walking unnatural and effortful, seemingly without any deliberate simulation, even when there is nothing wrong with their muscles or nerves. Sometimes patients experience persistent pain or dizziness or can speak only in a whisper, without there being any identifiable physiological cause, even after months or years of medical investigations. The ways in which patients present are as plentiful as the number of symptoms.

When I treat such patients, I acknowledge that these illnesses, even if they have no clear-cut physical cause, are not made up or simulated; they are as real as any other illness, even if their cause is believed to be psychological.

It is difficult to know why an individual will have a particular symptom—for instance, paralysis rather than dizziness or speaking in a whisper. Back in the early 1900s, some psychiatrists believed that an individual's symptoms carried a symbolic significance. For example, someone who witnessed an appalling event might develop blindness. Although this sort of belief is still occasionally mentioned in psychiatry textbooks, not many people believe it.

In Roland's case, his symptoms began with a cough and a sore throat, but his persistent focus on his breathing developed into a preoccupation. His cousin told him that he must have been cursed, an idea that Roland felt was being fulfilled in the shape of serious illness. This worry served only to perpetuate his symptoms, until coughing and exhaling noisily through his nose was as natural to him as breathing. Such presentations are often known as "conversion disorders," referring to the theory that psychological stresses are "converted" into physical symptoms, although it should be acknowledged that there is little consensus on what such presentations should be called. Our disorganized classification system is a reflection of the different ways in which people have understood these symptoms over the years. Some diagnoses, such as conversion disorder, stem from the theory of Freudian psychoanalysis, while other diagnoses, such as "persistent physical symptoms," are descriptive, yet both might be talking about the same thing. The term "functional disorder" is commonly used to indicate that while the structures of the body—the nerves, muscles, and organs—are all intact, their function is impaired. Sometimes the terms used are pejorative or insulting (a "heart-sink patient," referring to the effect they have on a doctor's morale; a "fat folder," used to describe the thickness of a patient's notes), and yet others such as "supratentorial" (pointing to a region of the brain), while respectful and medical-sounding, suggest that the cause lies in the brain and are a wink to fellow professionals that the doctor thinks it is all psychiatric.

As I dictated my letter to Roland's GP, I picked up his file and two letters fell out. The first was from an ear, nose, and throat (ENT) specialist, who had diagnosed a problem with his vocal cords. The second was from a neurologist, who had diagnosed a disorder of the nervous system. I began to worry. Had I completely misread the situation? I wondered whether to commit my diagnosis to the notes, my confidence in it steadily waning. I knew the ENT and neurology consultants to be sharp and capable doctors, not the sort who were casual about diagnoses. My diagnosis seemed even less sound when Roland came back to see me some weeks later, smiling and relieved that his symptoms had all but gone. It turned out that, lacking any confidence in his trio of physicians, he had laid out all his cares to a sympathetic priest, who agreed with him that he must have been cursed and administered holy water, thereby effecting this miraculous cure.

I felt chastened. Roland had seen four "healers," each of whom had reached a conclusion based on our understanding of the human body or mind. We had all seen what we wanted to see: the ENT specialist found a problem with the vocal cords, the neurologist found a problem with his nerves, the psychiatrist found a problem with his mind, and the priest with his soul. I found this unsettling; I had always believed that the way I saw things was the way that they were.

Medicine is narrow like that; we tend not to question our beliefs. In all medical textbooks, there is a formula for presenting an illness. It starts with epidemiology (how common the illness is), the etiology (what is considered its cause), its presentation (how the illness looks to the doctor), its course (what the natural history of the illness might be if it is left untreated), and its prognosis (outcome). Treatments that alter the natural prognosis are discussed, and Man triumphs over Nature.

I have taught medical students in teaching hospitals throughout my career; they believe that all symptoms are the product of a disease, which should be investigated and a cure offered. This process becomes second nature to medical students during their training and therefore goes unchallenged. There is an implicit belief that anything else is not real medicine. When I try to teach them a different way of thinking, they at first look slightly skeptical and then unsettled. I explain to them that symptoms are part of life and that most of the time, tiredness, pain, dizziness, or backache don't indicate any disease at all. Good doctors realize this, and a significant part of their role is to judge which symptoms to investigate and which to ignore. But mainstream medical thought and public opinion disagree with my hypothesis; symptoms are seen as indicative of illness, based on the prevalent infectious disease model of medicine that is practiced in the West.

In this model, an infectious agent is identified, an antibiotic or other cure is developed to attack the infectious agent, and a cure is effected. Treatment of infectious disease was the first major success of modern medicine, as dogma and superstition began to be replaced by a more evidence-based approach. That purely scientific model has had great success in many areas of medicine. It has helped in the understanding and treatments of cancers, heart disease, and kidney disease, to name just a few. It is for this reason that it has become the only game in town for the past several decades.

Yet to focus solely on the scientific aspects of illness, paying no attention to the social aspects, is a mistake that we continue to make. After all, this approach will not tell us which patients will ignore their symptoms or neglect their treatment, who will change their lives to improve their outcome, whose family will support them, which patients will develop depression and long for the end, and who will find a resilience they did not know they had. In other words, understanding the science of an illness often tells you little about how successful the treatment of an individual will be.

It gets worse. This scientific approach to the practice of medicine leads to countless unnecessary investigations. Eventually, when all these don't reveal much, the patient's symptoms are dismissed as imaginary. Sometimes a dreaded "incidental finding" that has nothing to do with the symptoms you were investigating shows up on a blood test or scan, thus opening up a whole new front in overinvestigation and overtreatment. For patients like Roland, the problem is not that their symptoms are not real—they are—but that they are not caused by the sorts of pathology that you read about in medical textbooks.

We usually don't think much about what health actually *is*, but rather instinctively judge whether we are in good health. When we do think about it, it is generally in "biological" terms—whether our organs are doing what they ought to. Yet good health, rather than simply meaning that your organs are all functioning correctly, is a subjective feeling of well-being influenced by a huge number of factors. The idea that closer scrutiny of our bodies will improve our longevity or general health is a fallacy; in fact, quite the opposite is true. As Benjamin Franklin astutely observed, "Nothing is more fatal to health than an over care of it." We have yet to learn this lesson and are encouraged into an increasing number of screening programs, wellness checks, and initiatives to raise awareness, all of which has made us more worried about our health than ever, although we have never been so healthy. As Marcel Proust observed more than a century after Franklin, "For one disorder that doctors cure with drugs (as I am told they occasionally do succeed in doing) they produce a dozen others in healthy subjects by inoculating them with that pathogenic agent a thousand times more virulent than all the microbes in the world, the idea that one is ill."

When medical historians evaluate this period of our history, they will see it as the age of the self. Wearable devices measure the amount of sleep we get, our heart rate, and the number of steps we take each day, yet there is little evidence that such analysis improves our long-term health outcomes. It does, however, lead to hypochondriacal concerns in the vulnerable, whose good health is eroded by health anxieties triggered by their scrutiny of health data.

It is not just the vulnerable, though, who suffer from our preoccupation with health and well-being. Despite the falling mortality rates and improved treatments for disease in the West, we just don't seem to feel as healthy as previous generations did. One study that examined health trends over the second half of the twentieth century in the United States showed that for both short- and long-term medical conditions, people were sicker and more disabled than their forebears. Another study, again in the United States, observed that with a 10 percent increase in the population, the number of people permanently limited by disability increased by 37 percent. How can this be? How can there be such a sharp increase in the number of people disabled by illness? At least part of the explanation lies in our expectations of how we perceive and think about our health.

Consider back pain, a leading cause of disability. In the United States, low back pain is estimated to cost the healthcare system over $100 billion per year. Studies in Western countries have shown increasing rates of low back pain, an increase not easily explained by any increased incidence of back disease. The most likely explanation came from a German study, which compared the rates of back pain between East Germany and West Germany before reunification in 1990, until a decade after East Germany and West Germany were reunified. East Germany, formerly a communist country, had a rate of back pain at least 10 percent lower than West Germany before 1990. Over the course of the next ten years, East Germany "caught up," and by the end of the study, it had the same high rates of back pain as West Germany. The authors of the study had little doubt that beliefs and attitudes toward back pain, rather than any actual disease, had been transmitted from West Germany to East Germany and were likely to have resulted in the greatly increased rates of low back pain.

How then should we think about health? Why did East Germany and West Germany have such different expectations about back pain, so that the poorer East German population felt healthier than their wealthier neighbors in West Germany? Nothing changed in their backs over the next decade, yet East Germans began to feel this part of their anatomy to be more painful, with all the overprescription of pain medication, disability, and economic disadvantage that back pain brings. This is not illness as most people see it or how I imagined health problems when I was studying at medical school.

Health is not just the absence of disease, but something less concrete, more ethereal. It is a subjective feeling, not always easy to measure and subject to the vagaries of our mood and expectations. All of this is frustratingly unscientific and messy, a hinterland somewhere between medicine and mind. It is an area where many doctors prefer not to go, preferring instead the crisp certainties of a scan result, an X-ray, a surgical procedure.

As our scientific understanding of the body has deepened, there has been a fragmentation of medicine. It has split off into many different subspecialties, because there's simply too much for one person to know. The advantage is that there is a great level of expertise about each organ system in the body, and patients with disease in that part of their body get a high level of care. The downside is that many doctors don't know too much outside of their specialist area. This narrowed perspective has led to a loss of wisdom. It means that the delivery of healthcare is focused and technical, less likely to take into account other factors like patient personality or mental health, which significantly influence the presentation of symptoms. Here, the application of a technical approach to medicine is a disaster. Patients with symptoms that have nothing to do with disease end up having multiple investigations in a fruitless attempt to find the cause. It's like trying to open a door lock with the wrong key. Rattling the key around and trying harder and harder to turn it in the lock is an act of futility. It will never come to any good and usually will end up doing some damage. So it is with medicine.

For many patients we end up doing them no good at all, and we harm quite a few more through unnecessary medical procedures. We make patients of normal people who don't need to be in the healthcare system. That people do not respond to our disease-focused approach is seen as a failure of medicine, and our solution is usually to apply more of it. It *is* a failure of medicine, but not because we lack the technical abilities to understand the human body. It is a failure to understand people—why they develop symptoms, why they come to see a doctor—and often a failure to understand what they want from their interaction with healthcare.

One of the studies that I often think about in relation to the disconnect between health as it is experienced and measured involved people who were recovering from a heart attack. After a heart attack, the heart works less efficiently because some of its muscle has died; this is expressed as an ejection fraction, which refers to the amount of blood expelled from a heart's pumping chamber. A normal ejection fraction is over 55 percent, but after a heart attack, this figure will fall, dependent on the amount of damage. The researchers found the level of disability after a heart attack does not always relate directly to the ejection fraction, but surprisingly to patient beliefs about their illness. If someone believes that their illness will have serious consequences, their lives start to shrink, they stop exercising and having sex, and they live a much more sedentary life. By contrast, if people believe their illness can be controlled, they are more likely to attend rehabilitation programs, get on with their lives, and resume the work and activities they had previously enjoyed. It was their beliefs that determined the outcome and activity. Physical activity after a heart attack is protective. This remains true even when the damage caused by the heart attack is more significant—you can have an ejection fraction of 45 percent and be crippled by it, or an ejection fraction of 35 percent and lead a fulfilling life.

We know plenty about the body—its anatomy, physiology, pathology; the problem is that we—doctors and patients alike—play surprisingly little attention to the ways in which our emotions influence how we perceive our bodies and experience our health.

My own journey into psychiatry was a meandering one. I never planned to study medicine at university, but after years of parental pressure, I was eventually persuaded to apply. Although I had been born and raised in Britain, my parents had something of a second-generation immigrant's view of progress and thought that becoming a doctor would mean that I had finally arrived.

Medical school interviews are a strange process. It is widely considered to be the kiss of death to say, when asked why you are applying, that you "want to help people." This was seen as a trite and superficial answer, whether it was true or not, and I knew to avoid saying it. I can recall only one boy in my year saying it at his interview, and he was met with the terse reply, "Well, why don't you study nursing, then?" I'm glad I was never asked the question, as I knew that "My parents made me apply" wasn't a great answer, either.

If I was asked now why I am interested in medicine, my answer would be "Because I am interested in people," though it would never have occurred to me during my time at medical school that this was relevant. Back then, the emphasis was on medicine as a science. We learned the anatomy of humans, dissecting corpses of people who had donated their bodies to "medical science." The smell of formaldehyde still transports me back to the old anatomy room, with its rows of dead bodies lying on the dissecting tables. By the start of my third term, when the anatomy demonstrator told a class of students to "Go and get yourselves a leg to dissect," I was so desensitized to it that I didn't think twice about ambling over to a large bucket at the back of the room and fishing out a human leg, taking care not to accidentally hit somebody with it on the way back to my desk.

But what do teenagers really understand about life and death, or the other important questions regarding our existence? I'm sure that's why far more students of psychiatry start their training as postgraduates. Medical school teaches a dispassionate and clinical analysis of disease on the human body. We learned about anatomy (where things are in the body), physiology (how the normal body operates), biochemistry (how cells work), neuroanatomy (dissecting human brains), neurophysiology (how a normal brain works), pathology (the study of illness and disease), and histopathology (looking at diseased bodies under a microscope), without once discussing the numerous ways in which changing the interaction with a patient can affect a health outcome.

Psychiatrists are all doctors and have received the same training at medical school as cardiologists, neurosurgeons, and general practitioners (GPs). We understand how the body works, what happens in disease, and how drugs both affect and are processed by the human body. But we also have something extra—an understanding of human nature, the product of an interest in people's lives, which is stimulated by seeing the myriad ways in which people's lives, personalities, intelligence, genetics, and misfortune can lead to different health outcomes and illnesses.

After I qualified as a doctor, the pressure of work was intense and the level of support was minimal; as a result, the more you came to see patients as clinical problems to be solved, rather than people with hopes, fears, and feelings, the easier life was. It was not uncommon for me to say to a colleague something like "I'll go and see the gallbladder in cubicle one while you see the hemorrhoids in cubicle four. Then we can review the overdose in intensive care." Nobody thought it odd that the patients' names often weren't used. But as the years passed, my humanity and curiosity about the anguish that might have led to such overdoses was slowly ebbing away. I became impatient and irritable and started to resent patients both for the trouble they were causing me and the sleep I was being denied. I felt as though I never left the hospital, and I grew deeply unhappy. I was single, which I blamed on being at work all the time, and increasingly cranky. I gained almost fifteen pounds over six months, undoubtedly a result of my diet of microwavable meals and bags of crisps eaten between shifts, supplemented by snacking on chocolates at the nurses' station.

One particular night on call made me realize how bad things had become. It was three A.M. and I had just dozed off, having been at work since eight the previous morning, when the bleep from my pager sounded. I was disoriented and initially thought it was morning, but when I picked up the message, I saw that it was from the hospital switchboard, which meant a caller from outside the hospital, which meant a GP, which meant an admission to Accident and Emergency

(A&E) in the next hour or so, which meant no sleep. I had a busy schedule the next day, so the prospect of another sleepless night made my shoulders sag. I answered the bleep, and the GP asked if I could accept a seventy-six-year-old woman with a suspected heart attack. It was not a request I could refuse, but I was graceless and cross.

After I put the phone down, I dozed fitfully, knowing I would soon be woken by the patient's arrival and alert to the sounds of the clanging hospital doors that drifted through the paper-thin walls. I must have dozed off again, because when the bleep sounded for a second time, I felt the same sense of bewilderment before I realized what was going on. The number on the pager was not from casualty to tell me that my patient had arrived; it was another outside call, which meant another patient. I dialed the number with a heavy heart before realizing that I was actually speaking to the original GP, who told me that the patient had died in the ambulance and would not be coming to casualty after all. Suddenly a night's sleep—or at least half a night—was back on. Euphoric, I turned off the light and sank back into the sagging hospital-issue mattress, but sleep would not come. I began to feel troubled by the realization that a human being whom I might have been able to help had died that night. I wondered whether she had had a family, retirement plans, responsibilities. My sense of contentment soon turned to shame; this was not who I was, nor who I wanted to be. I felt like I had lost my humanity, the most important quality a doctor can possess.

It took me several more years to get to psychiatry. The problem was that I found hospital medicine easy to manage—I had by then been elected as a member of the Royal College of Physicians, a British professional body for senior physicians within hospital medicine, and had risen to the grade below consultant—and it seemed somehow easier to keep going. But I was bored; after a few years, one heart attack looks pretty much like another, as do chest infections, kidney failures, arthritis, and many of the other problems I saw.

Overdoses were a different story. I would listen, transfixed, to the human dramas unfolding, appalled by the betrayals, sympathetic to the human failings, and astonished by the frequent banality behind tragic decisions. I remember one woman who was unhappy with her boyfriend's infidelities and her boring job, but it was only when she was in the bathroom at home, stooped over to pick up her hairbrush, and knocked her head on the underside of the sink that she decided to take an impulsive overdose. It seemed extraordinary that bumping your head on the porcelain sink might be the final straw. These stories drew me in and showed me a different side of life; I became aware of the fundamental failings and weaknesses that exist in us all.

Since changing careers to become a psychiatrist over twenty-five years ago, I have been able to do what I always really wanted: to listen to and understand ordinary people like you and me. I have heard the deepest fears and unrealized dreams of thousands of people, as well as their reactions to physical illness and their anguish at mental illness. I have come to understand that our similarities are much greater than our differences; I see and hear the same human reactions to love, loss, redemption, stress, and the development of mental illness. We are all scared, vulnerable, and uncertain. It is hard for us to admit this, even to ourselves. We like to exhibit our strength and confidence in all sorts of ways, as a means of asserting our success. We do it by the cars we drive, the vacations we take, the houses we live in, the clothes we wear, and our toned bodies, all of which are aimed at demonstrating our perfection and importance. But we do it because we are needy, uncertain, and underconfident. We crave the approval of others as a validation of our own lives, though deep down we want what everyone wants—to still the inner voice of criticism, to believe that we are good enough, and to know that our lives are worth something.

It is our personalities, attitudes, and beliefs that affect our lives at every stage. We all remember a classmate who could get away with anything at school, while less charming students could do no right. Some children progress effortlessly, while others struggle to make friends. People of average intelligence and talent can have great careers through hard work, persistence, and an occasional inflated sense of ability, while highly intelligent people can see their career stall, not realizing that they might sound argumentative or that their shyness may be seen as brusque. The myriad ways in which we interact with the world, whether verbally or nonverbally, all direct our path in life.

Similarly, our personality directly affects how we interact with our health. Do we ignore our symptoms or worry about every last physical sensation and visit the doctor repeatedly? Are we able to trust people, including doctors, or do we believe that Big Pharma is behind doctors' decisions and choose to ignore their advice? Perhaps we think the doctor has got it wrong or prefer to heed the advice we read on the internet or to emulate the behavior of friends who did the opposite of what they were advised. Perhaps you are so personable and persistent that the doctor wants to spend longer with you than with other patients, researching new treatments or even lobbying a pharmaceutical company for a particular drug. Religious or cultural beliefs may lead someone to think that their illness is a punishment. Depression can make someone feel that their treatment is pointless, to the extent that they don't seek treatment, while I have seen manic patients who believe that they are doctors making decisions regarding their treatment, with tragic consequences. Our beliefs, eloquence, expectations, charm, persistence, and mental health all significantly influence health outcomes, yet they are considered far less often than their importance would suggest.

The psychiatry I specialize in is at the intersection between mind and body. It draws on my early career working as a physician in internal medicine, as well as later in psychiatry, working in the community and inpatient psychiatry wards. For almost twenty years now I have been employed by a mental health trust to work in a general hospital. It is the sort of hospital most people have been in dozens of times, with the usual round of medical and surgical outpatients, inpatient wards, and operating schedules. People attend for their physical health problems, expecting the consultation to conclude with a diagnosis, a prescription, perhaps even an operation. Very few people going into a hospital believe that the outcome of their hospital appointment will be a visit to a psychiatrist, but for many of them, it transforms their care.

Health is complex. It takes an understanding of human nature, as well as an understanding of the body, to deliver effective care. There are difficult judgments to be made and uncertainties to acknowledge. One must be flexible and able to tolerate uncertainty. The human body can fail in a limited number of ways, but there are endless ways in which people's lives, experiences, personalities, and mental health can interact with their health and present to a doctor. This is an area to which I have always been drawn.

Exploring how personality and mental health dictate our experience of well-being is the subject of this book. It might seem hard to believe that our minds exert such an influence over our bodies, but it is true— they dictate all that we are, as well as all that we will become. Our minds shape the way we understand and react to symptoms that we develop, dictate the treatments we receive, and even influence whether the remedies will work.

What follows is a look at many of the problems that have brought patients to my clinics over the years. It will perhaps give you some understanding of what psychiatrists in a general hospital do. I write in the hope that you might learn to think in a new way about your mind, your body, and your health.

STIGMA

In the 1980s and 1990s, mental illness was very rarely discussed, and admitting to having a mental illness was regarded as shameful. It was one of those topics that were just never spoken about, similar to how much you earn or whether you're having an affair. Someone with mental illness would be discussed in scandalized tones over the garden fence. It's difficult to remember, now that everyone, including the British royal family, openly discusses mental illness, that we were once so uncomfortable with the subject.

I have long wondered about to what extent this newfound openness is a good thing. Having discussions about mental illness (usually referred to in the press as "mental health") certainly helps to reduce the shame and stigma of mental illness. Indeed, for most of history, mental illness was feared and sufferers were victimized. There is evidence that those who are unable to talk about their emotional problems, and particularly people who are socially isolated and lonely, are at higher risk of suicide. They are unable to unburden themselves of their problems and receive the help and support they need. We need to lose the notion that masculinity is about being strong and silent, or that mental illness is a sign of weakness. The more commonly and openly mental illness is discussed, the more normal it becomes.

On the other hand, the mental illnesses that are talked about are usually those that are relatively minor and sufficiently sanitized for public consumption. For example, while royalty may admit to experiencing sadness as a result of bereavement, I suspect that no member of the royal family would be encouraged to talk about their schizophrenia, hallucinations, or paranoia. This rather perpetuates the idea that some illnesses are still too stigmatized to talk about and that much of what is publicly discussed relates to more minor problems that straddle the boundary of normal human experience.

I think it might have been the Americanization of culture in the UK that allowed us to talk about emotions more openly. Who can forget (no matter how hard you try) the Jerry Springer style television talk shows of the 1990s, with their noisy and personal revelations? Situations that would have been a cause of deep shame in any other generation were now talked about openly, and even with some amount of pride.

I remember getting into a lift at the hospital with a mother and her grown-up daughter during that period. They had been arguing as I approached the elevator bank; I didn't gather the reason, but it seemed to be a fairly standard something-and-nothing kind of row. The doors opened and the three of us got in, but their argument simply carried on, without it occurring to either of them that I might feel awkward at having to listen to it or they might feel a measure of shame for such a carry-on. It seemed from the covert glances that they both gave me that they might even be taking a kind of pride in the argument. It felt to me like a demonstration of a change in social behavior and the adoption of new norms.

The *Big Brother* TV show and other reality television programs that followed have furthered such self-revelation, which has in some ways led to a more open and destigmatized society. We have replaced the traditional British and American value of tolerance with an insistent demand for acceptance and have thus come to accept both behaviors and people who are different from the conventional. Where this includes mental illness, it can only be a good thing.

This shift in attitudes was encouraged by Dr. Mike Shooter, president of the Royal College of Psychiatrists between 2002 and 2005. I remember listening, spellbound, as he gave a speech at a conference in 2002 about the onset of his depression. He described how it had begun while he was a medical student and explained how it had affected him. Speaking without notes, he created an intimate atmosphere and painted a vivid picture of the black veil of depression. I felt privileged to have been present at such a confessional moment.

Around this time it also became fashionable for former psychiatric patients, referred to as "service users," to sit on interview panels for the appointment of consultant psychiatrists. This led to a slightly uncomfortable situation at my first consultant interview. The interview began with one such service user asking why I thought I'd make a good consultant psychiatrist—standard interview fare, a lightly lobbed ball to be smashed to the boundary. It was the next question that caught me off guard, although perhaps I should have been expecting it. "Do you have any personal experience of mental illness?" I felt like I should help the interview process and a curt no didn't seem appropriate, but the question itself felt intrusive. After all, cardiologists would not be asked in a job interview whether they had ever had a heart attack. I wondered if our confessional climate had gone too far.

The question of whether I had any personal experience of mental illness reminded me of my childhood in Manchester. All my family lived there; the city had been the final destination for my great-grandparents after their flight from the pogroms and persecutions that had been inflicted upon the Jews in Europe. Among those relatives I had two great-aunts, Pearl and Sadie, who lived together in a detached house in Prestwich, North Manchester. They had spent all their adult lives in the house and had barely touched it since moving in, some time during the 1940s. We would visit them every Saturday afternoon, walking to get there through streets crowded with bearded men in black coats and hats, going to or from synagogue in the heart of suburban Jewish Manchester.

Sadie had last left the house in 1962, when she had attended my parents' wedding. When she was out of the house in her teens one day, she became faint and dizzy. She was overwhelmed with anxiety, and the dizziness went away only when she returned to the safety of home. From then on, each time she left the house, the dizziness and breathlessness returned, until she went out less and less, and her life gradually shrunk. She made one final effort—to attend my parents' wedding—before deciding that it would be easier if she didn't leave the house at all.

Sadie found things to do at home. She was a talented cook, so each Saturday afternoon my family would sit in the little oak-paneled snug, from where Sadie would pass fried fish, herring, pickles, and a variety of homemade cakes through the serving hatch that led to the kitchen. My siblings and I would sit drinking fizzy pop and eating cake, occasionally catching one another's eye as we removed long hairs from the middle of the slices. After tea, while the adults continued to chat, we would move to the living room and fight over who would get to sit on the burgundy velour Parker Knoll reclining chair with built-in footrest. We'd then settle down to watch the wrestling on *World of Sport*, followed by *Doctor Who*. The carpet in the living room, patterned with cocktail glasses, wouldn't have looked out of place on a 1940s cruise ship. The difficulty came when one of us needed to use the toilet; we got so worked up about the quiet, creepy feel of the upstairs of the house that we were too frightened to go alone. The three of us had a deal that we would always go in pairs, with one of us standing guard outside the toilet door while the other quickly had a pee.

As Great-Aunt Sadie never left the house, she had a dog to keep her company, though because she never left the house, neither did the dog. Brandy was a mongrel with a clump of hair that dangled over his backside. The only time he would become animated was when the doorbell rang or when someone attempted to cut this terrifically ugly clump of hair with a pair of scissors. For years, he ambled around, the matted hair swinging from side to side over his rump like a pendulum. Sadie adored Brandy and could not do enough for him, but although the dog was fed the choicest cuts of meat, his was a gilded cage. The extent of his world was where he could get to on the end of a length of clothesline tied to his collar—he could amble around the front garden, but no farther.

In time, deprived of other canine company, Brandy became withdrawn and slightly unhinged. When he finally died, he was replaced by a poodle called Mij (named after its original owner Jim, but spelled backward), a frisky little thing that would try to hump your leg when you sat down. I fear that the confinement also made Mij mentally unbalanced. As a teenager, I began to wonder if dogs could get mental illness in the same way that humans do, and whether that may account for a docile pet's becoming moody and, unable to articulate its distress in any other way, biting the postman.

But while her dogs were a pleasant distraction, the reality was that Sadie spent her whole adult life indoors because of agoraphobia. If someone had been sentenced to house arrest for life, there would be an outcry, and yet this was the sentence Sadie had imposed upon herself. She missed all the normal milestones of life—getting a job, finding a partner, perhaps having children. But as well as the milestones, she also missed out on the everyday details that make up a life. She missed the glance exchanged with a fellow passenger on a bus, the small talk at the supermarket checkout, the smoky smells of autumn, a drive at night with just the right song on the radio, freshly mown grass on a summer afternoon—a whole lifetime of experiences, both big and small. Since her last experience of life beyond her little house was in 1962, everything she knew about the outside world came from television and the radio. And all of this was the consequence of agoraphobia, a mental illness often considered minor and inconsequential, nothing like schizophrenia or "serious mental illness." Yet it devastated her life in a way that very few other illnesses would have.

The sideboard in Sadie's living room was always stacked with formulaic Mills & Boon romance novels, churned out so that there was a new one each month. The medical romances in the series were identified by an ECG trace in the corner of the front cover, the familiar wave form of the heart's electrical activity also indicating the palpitating intoxication of romance. In these novels, a handsome-but-arrogant doctor would fall under the spell of a beautiful-but-caring nurse and be seduced not only by her beauty but by her essential goodness. And if your only experience of romance is Mills & Boon and you don't have real life to fall back on, you can end up believing that it's real. So Sadie lived these novels, in a similar way that people can now live in their own computerized virtual reality. Years later, after Sadie had a stroke, she was delirious for a few weeks. Conversations with her drifted between the here and now and a fantasy world; she would often talk of a tall, dark, handsome stranger who was coming to take her away. It broke my heart.

Sadie's sister Pearl had been overweight all her life, but over the years she seemed to get steadily bigger. She went to work each day in the family business, a furniture shop in Rochdale, and brought an income to the house, while Sadie did all the cooking and housework.

Just like Sadie, Pearl never married and would never see a doctor—

the latter was a principle that she repeated frequently and loudly. Where that came from was unclear, although I suspect it had something to do with her self-consciousness about her weight. As a child, she would hide in a cupboard whenever the doctor paid a house visit. Perhaps in those days, doctors were more judgmental and would have highlighted her weight problem unsympathetically. As a result, she would not see a doctor for any problem, big or small.

Once Pearl was an adult, any attempt to request some form of rationalization for such an extreme position was met with the stubborn repetition of the same phrase, "I don't see doctors," followed by a jutting out of her chin and the end of the discussion. So she never discussed her weight with a doctor, or the reddish-brown marbling on her shins (from sitting too close to the electric heater, something that Sadie had, too, and that I later at medical school discovered was called erythema ab igne).

A sequence of events eventually forced Pearl to become housebound, too. The first was the unionization of the workforce in the furniture store, which encouraged the store workers to make demands of the management, and to assume that any resistance represented the usual story of the bosses trying to oppress the workers. Unfortunately for everyone concerned, Pearl and the family had not been exaggerating, and the workers' increasing demands helped bankrupt the business. Eventually it folded, putting everyone out of a job, including the salesmen, the foreman, the cashiers, and Pearl.

While this was going on, with the stress starting to tell, Pearl had an accident on the way home from work. She tripped on a raised curb, fell onto the road, and was too big and in too much pain to get up. She refused an ambulance ("I don't see doctors") and was eventually helped from the street into a car and taken home. Too badly shaken by the incident to risk another episode, she would never again venture outside.

On the Saturday afternoons we spent at their house, my enduring memory of Pearl is of her large hands holding the teapot, palms and fingers flat on the surface. Nobody else could touch it because it was far too hot, though Pearl didn't seem to feel the scalding heat. She spoke in a distinctive raspy voice as the week's events were dissected, while I kept glancing at the door, waiting for my chance to claim my place on the recliner for *World of Sport* and *Doctor Who*.

I always felt guilty when we left Pearl and Sadie's house. They were both incredibly generous to us, and I felt their kindness and love, even though as a child I was unable to articulate a response. Until we saw them the following weekend, I would go to school and my parents to work, all of us interacting with the outside world, while they would see only the inside of their house. When it was time to go home, I would kiss their whiskery cheeks, noting Pearl's strangely soft peaches-and-cream complexion, and accept the five-pound note they pressed into my hand before dodging the yapping dog and jumping into the car home. I would then have my regular Sunday game of football the next day, followed by the gathering melancholy of a Sunday evening, with a week of school looming.

After Sadie died, Pearl became increasingly immobile but still resisted any medical intervention. Her life steadily shrunk, with her bedroom now moved to the downstairs front room, which still resonates in my memory with the Seder nights of my childhood. Eventually, the situation became unmanageable, and hospital admission was unavoidable. It was at that point that Pearl was discovered to have an underactive thyroid gland. I was by then a medical student, and everything started to make sense: her weight, her peaches-and-cream complexion, her perpetually hoarse voice, and even her sparse eyebrows were all well-known effects of an underactive thyroid. The solution was simple: one tablet of thyroxine to replace the hormone, taken daily, was all she needed.

So my great-aunts, now lying next to each other in a cemetery in

North Manchester, had the course of their lives altered by what would today be considered minor health problems. Sadie's agoraphobia confined her to a lifetime indoors but would have been a treatable condition, if only she had sought help. And if Pearl had been able to get over her irrational distrust of doctors, she would have received her daily thyroxine tablet and lived a life without the disadvantages of untreated hypothyroidism.

There we have it: two lives defined and constrained by a reluctance to seek help for what would be considered minor and treatable health problems. I don't know whether a failure to seek medical help should be considered a mental health problem of its own, but when people think of life-dominating health problems, they probably think of illnesses such as cancer, kidney failure, or multiple sclerosis rather than of Pearl and Sadie.

I had no idea how to convey my sense of melancholy and despair at what might have been during my first interview to be a consultant. How could I do justice to the mix of emotions and to my enduring childhood memories of the constant presence of Pearl and Sadie, two brave, kind, and generous people whom I loved? I didn't feel I could, and I wasn't sure I really wanted to. However well-intentioned, the question about mental illness in my family had needled me. I gave some bland and formulaic type of interview response, perhaps stating the truth that mental illness is common and affects most families in one way or another, and I was not surprised when I learned that my application had not been successful.

Yet for a time after the interview, I kept thinking back to Pearl and Sadie. Why are some illnesses considered more important than others? I believe it comes from a perception that some illnesses can be safely ignored, the sufferers seen as sad or inadequate, rather than ill. Quiet, uncomplaining, and avoidant of attention, they want nothing so much as life to leave them alone, and the tragedy is that it does. Where are the advertising campaigns and lobby groups attracting research funds for the sorts of problems faced by Pearl and Sadie?

I was once on the board of a mental health charity, at a meeting where a Defeat Stigma campaign was being discussed. There was almost no discussion of people incapacitated by agoraphobias, social phobias, health anxieties, or obsessional behaviors, whose daily lives are a torment of self-doubt and lack of productivity, quietly suffering away from the glare of the latest health campaign. Maybe I was just being too impatient. Attitudes toward things like mental illness change over generations, not just a couple of years. Perhaps it will just take time, and the cumulative effect of many anti-stigma campaigns, for us to notice the difference.

CULTURE

I am often struck by how the culture in society seeps into the medical culture and plays such a part in how patients are treated and symptoms are investigated. How we view health and illness is a complex mixture of our current biological understanding and our cultural, philosophical, and religious beliefs. Back in the ancient world, at the time of Hippocrates, many of the same questions were being asked then as now, about how we define illness and health. The prevailing view back then was that many illnesses—for example, seizures and fits—were the product of possession or curses by the gods. Hippocrates, that great physician who gave his name to the Hippocratic Oath, argued against this view, and believed that illness was the consequences of a brain disorder, of the body having gone wrong. Hippocrates sought to modernize the understanding of medicine by setting out how illness related to the body, not to malign spirits.

In modern-day medicine, the debate about how the mind and body interact and influence each other is always referred back to René Descartes, the seventeenth-century French philosopher. It was Descartes's belief that the body comprised a physical entity—the nerves, muscles, blood vessels, and so forth—and an ephemeral spirit, the mind. He saw the mind as entirely separate from the body. The mind might have been able to communicate with the body via the brain, but it was not a part of the body. This separation of the mind and body has become known as Cartesian dualism.

The roots of dualism are religious, with an eternal soul both separate from and connected to the body. Yet in medicine it has come to mean the lack of connection between the mind and body in a clinical sense. The prevailing medical culture now sees the body as a machine, with organs in the body behaving in a predictable way. It follows that when things go wrong, when patients develop symptoms, that these will then be easily traced back to the organ or system at fault. But as Rick J. Carlson said in his 1975 book *The End of Medicine,* "To think of man as a machine does aid us in understanding something about bodily function and about man's role in the universe, but it does not follow that treating the body as a machine will heal it. But medicine appropriated the idea as the premise for its practice." This is the essence of the current culture. Our belief in science is almost absolute. It is hard for us to conceive that when symptoms occur, when people experience pain or fatigue or dizziness, that the symptoms can both be very real and yet not caused by any underlying problem with the body. This is so sharply at odds with the prevailing culture that it can be hard for both clinicians and patients to accept. The fact that this exact scenario is seen every day in clinics up and down the country is a bewildering and inconvenient truth, usually dealt with by being ignored. There is, in the words of the British philosopher Gilbert Ryle, a ghost in the machine.

Mostly we don't think about the culture we live in any more than a goldfish thinks about the water it swims in. It is often as much as we can manage to just keep up with the job that we do. In fact, the only emotion I experienced on my first day as a doctor was terror. I certainly wasn't thinking about the culture of medicine. The job gave little time for anything other than the relentless workload. In the 1990s, there was no induction to show you the ropes, no welcome to the hospital, no gradual easing in to get you up to speed. You simply started on August 1, and if that happened to be a Saturday, which in my case it was in 1992, you turned up to a new hospital you may never have visited before, someone handed you a pager, and . . . that was that. You were told to get on with it. The weekend meant being on call, dealing with emergencies from casualty or the wards, with a skeleton coverage throughout the hospital. There was, somewhere else in the hospital, a registrar with a few years of experience under their belt, someone who was invariably busy and always irritated by having a junior doctor bother them over decisions they considered trivial. So my first experience of being a doctor was being thrown into the deep end, with no welcome, no induction, nowhere to put my bag, nowhere to get lunch if I missed the 12:00–2:00 P.M. lunch period, and nowhere to get dinner past eight.

Even now, decades later, there is the same institutional indifference to doctors, and I ponder the truism that you cannot run two cultures in one organization. You cannot treat the medical staff (or any other staff, for that matter) badly and expect them to treat patients well. It simply doesn't work. Badly treated staff, resentful and unhappy, tend to pass those feelings on to the public whom they treat. This is not because they are bad people, but because they are stressed, sometimes underpaid, and often underappreciated. If the health and well-being of staff is not looked after, then the health of those patients that they are meant to be treating suffers, too. It takes an unusually farsighted chief executive to see this—although in their defense, they are usually themselves battling intolerable pressures from government or shareholders, and the misery gets passed downward.

On my first day as a new doctor, I had to locate my on-call room. I eventually found it on the second floor of a grim concrete building. Over the course of the next several years, as I moved jobs every six months, I became something of an expert on these rooms. Here was the prototypical on-call room: It always had a sagging mattress on the bed (rumor had it that they were condemned hospital mattresses). You couldn't sleep comfortably on them anyway, because they had broken springs and were thin and lumpy; you usually ended up rolling into the dip in the middle during the night. The mattress smelled of generations of anxious and unhappy trainees, who themselves had endured fitful and unrefreshing sleeps on it. The curtains over the windows were thin, and for some unknown reason, they were usually a color somewhere between dark orange and brown. Temperature regulation in the room was always poor. The rooms were either sweltering, with radiators on full blast that wouldn't switch off, or freezing cold, with wind rushing in through the poorly fitted windows, making the frames rattle and the cheap orange curtains flap about. The rooms themselves were mostly situated an inconvenient distance from the wards, and sometimes a long (and at night often dangerous) walk from the main hospital. In short, everything about the on-call room reflected the atmosphere of institutional indifference toward the junior doctors working in the hospital. But from a management perspective, this all made sense. What were you going to do about it anyway? You'd be gone in six months, and a new crop of frightened and demoralized juniors would take your place.

Nowadays, doctors don't have on-call rooms at all. These have become offices for various layers of management, a trend that was just beginning around the time that I qualified in 1992. On-call rooms are considered superfluous because of the changes in how medical care is structured. When I first became a doctor, like all my colleagues I was allocated to a "firm." This firm consisted of a consultant, and then in descending order of seniority, the senior registrar, registrar, senior house officer, and junior house officer. The firm became your family over the next six months. You spent nearly all your time with them (far more time than with any actual family you might have) and looked after "your" ward patients together. Every third or fourth night was spent with them on an on-call rota. Being on call meant arriving at work at eight A.M., working all that day and through the night, sometimes grabbing an hour or two of sleep in the on-call room, before working through the following day. It was tough at times (one week, I ended up working 140 hours because of various rota swaps), but it was with people you knew and trusted, and somehow going through it together eased the pain.

Junior doctors now work shifts that ostensibly give them a better quality of life, and it's true that they don't work quite the same number of hours. But the system is just as bad for the doctors, whose fractured rotas are the antithesis of good practice and consistent medical care. Of course doctors have always come low down on the list of hospital priorities, and the loss of the doctors' mess, of consultant dining rooms, and of the old "firm" medical structure, with a consultant working with and getting to know his or her team of juniors, has led to a lack of cohesion and loss of the esprit de corps that used to be so essential to morale.

Back then, psychiatry did not really enter the general hospital. There was a culture and a mindset that we were here to deal with physical health problems, and that was that. We did not have time for psychological aspects of illness. What we had was a conveyor belt of patients—a remorseless sea of faces, complaints, investigations, all of which allowed little time for thought. The priority was throughput, and speed was valued above almost everything. Psychiatrists working in the general hospital, with an interest in the overlap between physical and mental health, barely existed, and not at all outside the major centers and teaching hospitals. Frankly, it was easier not to ask about anything psychological, because there was nothing much you'd do with the information anyway. Patients themselves soon worked out that these aspects of their care did not seem particularly relevant to the doctors and would not volunteer them.

Deep down, I began to wonder whether ignoring psychological aspects of illness was a good idea. As I continued in hospital medicine and became more senior, I started to run outpatient clinics. Like everything else in medicine, you were just expected to turn up and know what to do without anyone telling you. Usually in the end, you'd gradually start to work it out. For each case in outpatients, you had to go back through the patient's file and construct a timeline of what had happened to them. This involved working out what symptoms the patient had presented with, what the findings were when they were examined, and whether your predecessors had come up with a list of potential diagnoses that they were considering (known in the trade as "differential diagnoses"). You then needed to work out what the doctors before you had done to investigate and resolve the problem.

Usually what the junior doctor would do, at least for any case that was difficult, was to kick the can down the road until they had moved on to a different department. This was accomplished by arranging a series of largely pointless investigations that achieved two main goals. First, it gave the appearance of activity, as though purposeless and unnecessary investigations were somehow a replacement for thoughtful analysis and clear decision-making. And second, it gave the patient the impression that their complaint was being taken seriously and thoroughly investigated. Yet even a first glance at the notes would often reveal that the patient's physical health complaints were being driven by stress, unhappiness, depression, or a variety of other psychological and social factors. This could be seen in the references to complex family dynamics, financial strain, mood and anxiety disorders. But by that point there was too much water under the bridge. The doctors had become too invested in the physical, and the patient believed it, too, sure that the doctors wouldn't keep looking for physical problems unless they expected to find them. It became easier to join your predecessors and evade the conversation that needed to be had, about whether your patient's physical problems could in fact be a reflection of psychological or social pressures. You just had to think of a couple more investigations that hadn't yet been done or repeat a couple that had. By the time all the investigations had come back, it would be the turn of the next doctor, and no longer your problem.

If my switch from medicine and into psychiatry had a pivotal moment, then it was here. It came with the dawning realization that medicine is being practiced in a way that, for many of the people it purports to help, worsens their physical health. This is done without malice, indeed with the best of intentions, as with most calamities. Consider the facts. In one well-known study carried out in primary care in the United States, of over 550 new complaints of common symptoms (such as chest pain, fatigue, dizziness, headache, back pain, numbness), an underlying physical cause was shown in only 16 percent of the cases. This is an eye-popping figure, meaning that in nearly all cases of people visiting their doctor with common physical symptoms, there's rarely a cause found and nothing for the doctor to treat. In this study, the doctor attempted treatment in just over half the cases, and often that was ineffective. Studies like this have been replicated since, and always with the same finding. A substantial proportion of problems presenting to the medical profession are not "medical" in the way that most people think about it. Most symptoms don't arise from a diseased organ in the body, yet we persist in pretending that they do.

Even if a patient makes it through primary care and gets to see a hospital specialist, because of chest pain, pelvic pain, tiredness, dizziness, bowel problems, or a variety of other ailments, the statistics look little better. A study carried out in London found that if you made it to a gynecology clinic, only 34 percent of symptoms could be explained medically by the specialist seeing you, with 66 percent having no medical explanation. In the neurology clinic it was not much better, with only 38 percent of patients having symptoms that the neurologist could explain. The same was true in gastroenterology (42 percent) and cardiology, where only about 45 percent of symptoms were thought to be explained by organic disease. For rheumatology, the figures were 55 percent, and for chest clinic, 60 percent. In a study carried out in a medical outpatient clinic in Holland, just 48 percent of outpatient attendees had a definite medical explanation for their symptoms.

Medically unexplained symptoms are expensive, too. All those unnecessary investigations add up, and in the UK are estimated to cost over £3 billion per year, which is close to 3 percent of the whole annual budget for the National Health Service. Sometimes the justification used for carrying out tests that doctors deep down know are going to tell them nothing is that they "reassure the patient." Interestingly, this is usually not the case. One study explored whether scanning patients with daily headaches would be reassuring for sufferers. On the face of it, it seems like a good idea. You can quickly disabuse patients of the notion that there's any serious cause for their headache, and they can get on with their life. Yet the results were disappointing. After one year, any relief the patient may have experienced after a normal scan had evaporated, as if the scan had never happened.

From time to time, policy documents are written that highlight the costs of medically unexplained symptoms. The costs are of course financial, in terms of unnecessary investigations (and the economic loss of unproductive patients unable to work); but just as important is the human cost of misapplying a medical framework to what is essentially a psychological problem. Reports are produced and statistics are presented; occasionally there is even a brief flurry of media interest. Yet the reports are soon forgotten, and medical practice continues entirely unchanged.

Michael Sharpe, a professor of psychological medicine at Oxford, together with his colleague Monica Greco, a professor at Goldsmiths, University of London, draws a distinction between illness and disease.

Illness is the patient's own subjective experience of symptoms, what they are suffering with. *Disease* is what the doctor diagnoses through investigations. Disease can be picked up on scans, in blood work, and on physical examination. Diseases are seen as "real" and objectively verifiable. Illnesses, though, are just a collection of symptoms, not validated by a disease label given by the doctor. For this reason, illness without disease is often seen as not "real," because nothing has shown up on the investigations. The patient's suffering is seen as suspect, their predicament a kind of moral failing. Say a person goes to their doctor complaining of dizziness. The doctor investigates, finds nothing abnormal, and says to the patient: "It's all good news. The investigations are entirely normal. You'll be relieved to know there's nothing wrong with you." Now the patient continues to suffer, but without the legitimacy of a disease. For the patient, the lack of findings on the tests is anything but good news. Colleagues and family may begin to question whether their suffering is genuine. Well-meaning (or not so well-meaning) people may advise the individual to "pull yourself together" and get back to work. When a patient has an illness with various troubling symptoms but no underlying disease to account for these, he is no longer seen as suffering, but rather as weak-willed, a person lacking moral fiber.

In this context, the medical model as it is currently employed, although failing many patients and hugely costly, makes some kind of sense. The countless rounds of investigations are an attempt to legitimize patients' suffering by giving them a disease label, thus absolving them of any blame for their illness. In societies where moral judgments are made of people, a psychological cause of illness, a diagnosis in which no disease is found, can be judged as blameworthy and shameful—even where the suffering is considerable. By contrast, illness caused by disease is seen as blameless, worthy of sympathy and societal support. Medicine fulfills the function of legitimizing illness because as a society, this is the role we have chosen for it.

This body-as-machine medical model is also maintained by an increasingly risk-averse culture. This aversion to risk means that, more than anything else, doctors fear missing a diagnosis, far more than they fear the harms of overinvestigation. Missing a diagnosis is the stuff of malpractice nightmares. On the other hand, overinvestigation is seen as perhaps a little overcautious, but generally a form of good medical practice. This is despite it being well known that overinvestigating symptoms can lead to very real harm, because no investigation is perfectly accurate or perfectly safe. Biopsies can miss the target, blood vessels can be punctured, little blobs of uncertain significance can appear on scans, equivocal blood test results can be returned from the laboratory. All of these lead to further anxiety for the patient, and almost inevitably further tests.

I can think of several patients I have seen in the past few years whose lives were all but ruined by a series of well-meaning doctors trying to explain every last detail of their presentation. One young man I was referred in my outpatient clinic had seen consultants in six different specialties (cardiology, rheumatology, neurology, autonomic nervous system, gastroenterology, ENT) before seeing me, in an attempt to explain some dizziness he had experienced. It was obvious to me, as surely it would have been to the other doctors, that what he had was an anxiety disorder, and the dizziness was the result of overbreathing, which commonly happens in anxious patients. Yet none of the specialists had felt confident enough to say this with certainty without first investigating whether his dizziness may after all have an underlying physical basis. For the best part of eighteen months, his life had been on hold. He was investigated for inner ear disease, balance disorders, low blood pressure, neurological causes, cardiac causes, damage to the nerves controlling blood vessels. He had endured X-rays, brain scans, blood tests, tilt tables. He had worn cardiac monitors for days at a time, had had dyes injected into blood vessels, had started on a treatment that made him both nauseated and exhausted. In light of his failing health, he had delayed getting engaged to his girlfriend, and work was what he did between hospital appointments. He had been subjected to more tests and scans than I could count (and I usually do count). He had experienced what is known as iatrogenic harm—in other words, harm caused by doctors.

When I first saw him, he was difficult to engage in conversation. He was in his twenties, youthful looking, although wary, and even a little guarded. He told his story in a formulaic way, because he had told it so many times before. The only time he perked up a bit was when I asked him if his experiences had made him mistrustful of doctors. The question seemed to have unlocked something. He told me that he had lost all confidence in the medical profession. Doctors had subjected him to so much discomfort and taken so much of his time, yet he was far worse off than when he began. On this point, I found it hard to disagree. He had been brought up to be respectful of authority and didn't like to challenge the doctors' opinion. I asked him how I would know if he was able to trust my opinion. He wasn't too sure about that, but again something in him softened. He was frightened and seemed desperate to talk about his fears and uncertainties, whether he was seriously ill or one of the worried well. The investigations had served only to heighten his fears of a serious illness, and his being passed from one specialty to another was exhausting.

I was direct with him, telling him that his problems were nothing more and nothing less than an untreated anxiety disorder, exacerbated by the ongoing health uncertainties and the investigations and treatment. After a long discussion, I could see that he was considering this, and in the end, he decided to go along with my formulation of his problems. And most gratifyingly, after starting treatment for his anxiety disorder with a single anti-anxiety medication, he was improved in four weeks and back to normal after eight weeks; I discharged him from my clinic shortly after that. The past eighteen months had been a nightmare he wanted to put behind him. Yet his case lingered in my mind. It was a demonstration of perhaps the biggest problem of all in our current risk-averse culture. All these rounds of investigations that patients are routinely subjected to means that doctors end up looking in all the wrong places for disease, meanwhile delaying treatment that can actually help the patient.

A colleague in the chest clinic referred another case to me just a few weeks after this. The referral was for a middle-aged woman with asthma that was causing breathing difficulties far in excess of any objective clinical findings. In other words, the asthma team had begun to suspect a psychological component to her illness. It seemed a fairly straightforward case. Being at that time relatively new to the hospital, I was eager to make a good impression on my consultant colleagues in the general medical clinics. In truth, I was finding it a lonely furrow to plow, being the only psychiatry consultant in a venerable old hospital like Guy's. Former Guy's physicians are famous throughout the medical world. They are immortalized on the wards named after them. Astley Cooper, the anatomist who gave his name to Cooper's testis, Cooper's ligaments of the breast, and Cooper's hernia, among many others; James Blundell, who performed the first ever blood transfusion; Richard Bright, who pioneered the study of kidney disease; Thomas Addison, who gave his name to the disease that the U.S. president John F. Kennedy later suffered with. There were centuries of history in the corridors. I felt like the reputation of psychiatry was on my shoulders. Determined to do a thorough job, I asked my secretary to see if the patient who had been referred, Margaret, had any psychiatric records. Back then, we had different sets of paper notes. One set of notes was for physical health, and the other, kept in an entirely separate location in the hospital, were the psychiatric notes. (Things have advanced since then. Now we have electronic notes, one system for physical health records, and the other, entirely incompatible system, is for psychiatric notes. Inevitably, the two systems do not talk to each other, and my junior doctors spend a proportion of their time typing into one set of notes, then emailing themselves the entry they just made, before logging into another notes system and pasting exactly the same entry there.)

A couple of days later, Margaret's notes had arrived from the medical records department. It was a thick sheaf, predictably with way too many letters and notes. As soon as I opened the notes, the whole thing burst open and pieces of paper slid out of the folder and onto the desk and floor. I bent down to retrieve the letters. The first letter I picked up was written using a typewriter, on a sheet as thin as cigarette paper. The letter was dated from the 1960s, and amid the yellowing margins and uneven typeface, the occasional word had been crossed out and corrected in ballpoint pen. It was from Margaret's primary school to her parents, advising them that their child's anxiety was impacting her school attendance and educational attainment. Next to it lay another letter from the school, briefer but otherwise identical, regretting that they had not received a reply to their previous correspondence. Other letters had fallen underneath my desk. These were from the 1970s and written in the high-handed language of doctors of a bygone era. Patients in the 1970s were not allowed to see their medical records (in fact patients would not have the right to see their medical records for another thirty years), so they were written with little consideration for how the patient might feel if he or she was to read what was in them. I picked up one of the letters from a physician, which was addressed to a long-since retired psychiatrist. "This girl [although she was by now twenty-one] came to see me complaining of chest pain, which she is concerned may be related to her heart. She came to see me in my outpatient clinic with a newspaper article about cardiomyopathy. I have to say, I found her theories rather fanciful. I explained this to her, and have discharged her back to your care."

Elsewhere on my desk, a psychiatric report written for the court had landed. Dated from the 1980s, it appeared that Margaret had been caught shoplifting. The report said she had taken some items from a pharmacy without paying. Her defense was that she had intended to pay, but a panic attack had overwhelmed her and she had bolted from the shop without stopping. The psychiatrist writing the report was sympathetic and considered her story plausible. I picked up handfuls of other letters, although they were by now hopelessly out of sequence, and I couldn't find out what had happened to her in court. I eventually started shoving the loose pieces of paper back into the folder. Some were near-illegible notes that had been written during her clinic appointments. I could make out brief snatches of prose written in a spidery handwriting, including "tense, agitated, inc. anxiolytic Rx," which broadly translated as some sort of justification for increasing her anti-anxiety medication because of ongoing symptoms. I couldn't help thinking that life for doctors was much simpler back then. A few scrawled notes, perhaps a prescription, and grateful and uncomplaining patients.

The physical health records were equally revealing. By the age of thirty, Margaret must have visited about half the medical departments in the hospital. She had had several invasive procedures, which all seemed to have generated side effects and ongoing pain, all of which were in turn reinvestigated. She had fallen down the rabbit hole of medical care. Strangely, though, this was where she wanted to be. She was entirely unresisting of the endless round of investigations, secure in the embrace of the medical profession. She had become a professional patient, steadily building her life around medical appointments.

I don't know what I was expecting when I finally met Margaret, but what was most notable about her was that in almost every respect, she was entirely unremarkable. She wore stonewashed denim jeans, sneakers, and a shapeless bottle-green shirt. Her thin shoulder-length hair was starting to gray. She spoke coherently, although there was a hint of anxiety in her voice, and one could sense her desperation to make a good impression. She told me a bit about her early childhood, most of which I already knew from the notes. She had grown up in a working-class family in a suburb of London and had always been an anxious girl. Her father worked on the railways, and her mother had never worked. In part this was because she was looking after her three children, and in part because of various ailments, including migraines, dizzy spells, and joint pains that kept her in bed for days at a time. Margaret's mother would often keep her out of school, as she had begun to develop abdominal pain when she was feeling under stress.

When she was sixteen, she developed appendicitis. After years of abdominal pain and absences from school, she had a hard time getting anyone to take it seriously. She said that her initial complaints had been dismissed by the doctors. It was only after her appendix had ruptured that the system clicked into gear, and she was soon taken to the operating theater. She recalled the event clearly, saying that afterward she began to have nightmares of dying in the hospital. She remembers becoming increasingly worried about her health, especially since "they didn't listen to me in the first place." This set the pattern for her future consultations with the healthcare profession. If anyone suggested that some of her symptoms might not be understandable in terms of organic illness, that perhaps they could be better understood as a reflection of her anxiety and preoccupation with her physical health, she would point to her previous experience. It was her trump card, the salutary lesson of what happens when doctors don't pay attention to their patients. And doctors, ever anxious not to be sued, fearful of missing something, always investigated.

It was obvious that her constant ill health was affecting her home life. She had by then married and had children, and after a brief time working for a textile company, her health problems curtailed any career. She rarely joined the family on holidays because of worries about being ill while she was abroad. Her constant series of ailments reminded me of one of those whack-a-mole stalls at a fair. As soon as one health problem had been resolved, another popped up somewhere else. And when there was no physical health problem, her anxiety would resurface and intensify. In this way, her life continued, an endless round of GP and hospital appointments and investigations. I wondered what would happen if she ever got well—what she would do with her life.

Over the years that she was my patient, she carried on in much the same way. At one level she understood what I was telling her about the link between mind and body and my explanation of her symptoms. But every time she felt a twinge anywhere in her body, it was all forgotten. She would work herself up into a state, convinced that this time, unlike all the hundreds of times that had gone before, was going to be the fatal episode. This was going to be like her appendix all over again, trying to convince everyone that she was genuinely unwell. Once this decision was made, she would be crying with pain, moribund and desperate. And it was never very long before another set of investigations would be carried out. Usually the results of these would be normal, although sometimes a minor and inconsequential abnormality would be found. In the context of all of Margaret's anguish and emotion, treatment would be offered, and this on occasion had included surgery. And so it went. This was Margaret's life.

My achievements with her were modest. I encouraged her not to visit the doctor for every minor symptom. I explained to her a fact that is well known but little discussed: that symptoms are normal and common, and in nearly all cases do not indicate any disease. It was difficult to make much progress with Margaret. Yet it was an even harder job to discourage the physicians and surgeons from overinvestigating. They could see the point of what I was saying, they understood well enough the pattern of behavior that had developed, but they were fearful of missing something, and ultimately it cost them nothing to investigate.

Investigating her always seemed like the safe option, even if it was not the right option.

I looked after Margaret for ten years. She had developed an unshakable belief that I had saved her life. I could never really work out why she thought that. Perhaps it was because I had seen her through a number of crises over the years. Usually her crises related to her receiving letters from officialdom, events that always threw her into a panic. Sometimes it was a family crisis or event. It was not hard to predict that an episode of anxiety or the development of a new symptom would follow.

Every December I would receive a card from her, accompanied by something she had made in an arts and crafts class—an oversize clay apple one year; the following year something that reminded me of Thor's cup, a kind of huge drinking horn. One year it was an enamel elephant. Eventually, with much emotion and drama, she moved to a different area, and I handed her care over to another psychiatrist. For all her insistence that I was the only reason she was alive, to me, her case seemed only to support my theory that the people I have done the least for are often the most grateful. I had done my best to keep her away from unnecessary medical investigations and treatments, focusing on improving her mental health. Yet at each turn I was undermined by a medical culture that struggles to cope with Margaret's kind of presentation, unaware that she represents the majority of people with health problems. I didn't blame anyone. Her doctors were all diligent and well-intentioned practitioners, and I suspect that they must have had their doubts about the wisdom of some of their investigations and the surgeries they subjected her to. It's just that they were constrained by a system of medical practice that is risk-averse and rigid. It is a culture in which the safe option is nearly always to overinvestigate. It struggles to accommodate patients like Margaret, the collateral damage in our relentless pursuit of disease.

MELANCHOLIA

I'm used to the reactions now when people discover I am a psychiatrist. Probably the commonest question is "Are you analyzing me now?," to which my reply is usually no (although occasionally "Yes, I noticed you scratching your nose just now when you asked . . .") but which belies a fundamental misunderstanding of how psychiatry works and what it is. We do not have our patients lie on couches and we don't ask them to free-associate. We do not know people's innermost thoughts just by watching them. We are not mind readers. I have never opened a consultation with the words "Tell me about your childhood." I do, however, find myself on an average day asking an extraordinary number of questions, and many of these are very personal.

It may surprise you to know that, despite the hundreds of "funny" birthday cards showing a psychiatrist's office with a patient lying on a chaise longue and a bearded psychiatrist seated on a chair at the head end, Sigmund Freud is barely mentioned anymore in medical school, let alone taught. Insightful though he was, Freud, who lived from 1856 to 1939, is a fading figure of a bygone era. He had some interesting things to say, of course. Freud developed the idea that inside every person's mind there was an id, a seething caldron of desires that provided the motivation for individuals, driving them forward, like the engine of a car. And like a car with an engine but no brakes, it wouldn't be long before there was a disaster. He therefore hypothesized that there was an opposite force, the superego, to act as a brake. He saw the superego as a harsh and restrictive set of moral rules, usually derived from parents or other authority figures, which were the standards that individuals needed to hold themselves to. Balancing the id and the superego was the ego, the conscious and self-aware part of ourselves. The ego directed our behavior in a socially acceptable way, navigating a course between our base desires on the one hand and our conscience on the other.

Freud's idea was to make the unconscious (id and superego) available to the conscious mind, and in doing so, we would come to know and understand ourselves. He believed that this greater self-awareness would effect the cure for whatever mental anguish we were trying to contend with. He gave his name to what are now called Freudian slips. These are slips of the tongue, such as saying "I must marry him when the tickets arrive," rather than "I must remember him when the tickets arrive." Freud thought these slips of the tongue revealed our innermost desires—in this case, a secret longing to marry the person. He also considered dreams to be of great significance. He believed that the subconscious mind, unhindered during sleep, was what led to dreams, and the interpretation of these was "the royal road to the subconscious." Freud thought that by these sorts of techniques he could access our deepest subconscious thoughts and desires. He hypothesized that this self-awareness was what we needed to overcome our psychological obstacles, and by understanding ourselves, we would be free of our neuroses.

The process of analysis in this way is lengthy. Individuals may be seen weekly, or even as often as five times per week. Trying to winkle out those unconscious memories, those repressed feelings and desires, is a time-consuming process. Progress is often measured in years, and the results in my view do not justify the considerable time and expense in undertaking therapies of this sort. And the prevailing view in modern psychiatry is that Freudian psychiatry is a phase that has run its course, one no longer considered relevant to day-to-day practice. The bell-bottomed jeans and scratchy beards of the 1970s psychiatrists have been replaced by the sober and sharper suits of the modern psychiatrist, with their MRI scanners and theories about mental illness as an autoimmune disease. Progress in clinical medicine is a path littered with ideas that have passed their prime. Some fade completely; others, such as psychoanalysis, lose their prominence but find a niche and don't quite disappear altogether.

One of the longest-standing ideas was the theory of the four humors, a hypothesis prevalent in medicine for 1,500 years, starting with the ancient Greeks. Back then, physicians did not specialize in different bits of the body, as they do today. In fact, as sociology professor and medical historian Andrew Scull points out in his book *Hysteria: The Biography,* to do so was the hallmark of quackery and amateurism. The prevailing view, one that lasted well over a thousand years, was that the mind and body needed to be in perfect balance. This balance was provided for by the four humors: blood, phlegm, black bile, and yellow bile (or cholera). The job of the doctor was to work out the way in which the sick patient had their humors misaligned, to correct the balance, and thus to provide the cure.

Depressed patients, according to this theory, had an excess of black bile. The Greek name for black bile is melancholia—hence the term "melancholy" that we use today. Manic patients had an excess of blood, causing excitable and explosive tempers. Prescriptions of bland and milky puddings became popular as a treatment in trying to dampen down the excess blood and to restore balance. Emetics to make patients vomit, bloodletting, and purging were all attempts to rebalance the humors.

The reason this theory lasted for well over a thousand years was that it was so elegant and explained everything: the workings of the body and our personalities, as well as the relationship between the body and the world around us. To give one example, phlegm was the humor associated with winter, thus providing an explanation as to why your nose would run in that season. The personality associated with phlegm was, unsurprisingly, phlegmatic. The theory appealed to our need for order and clarity. The theory of the four humors was based on an assumption, which in my experience is very rarely challenged, that things should make sense. Sometimes, as much in the world of quantum physics as in the world of emotions and psychiatry, they do not.

I was pondering all this in a clinic one Wednesday afternoon when I took the next patient into my consulting room. Simon was a successful lawyer, married with three young children, and had been prone to episodes of profound depression. It seemed to stalk him without reason or consideration of his circumstances, leaving him helpless and bereft. I thought back to a conversation I'd had some years previously as a junior doctor, having lunch with an eminent psychiatrist, discussing (as doctors sometimes do) what illnesses we would least like to have. His reply was instantaneous and unequivocal, and to me at that time surprising— severe depression. He said that while there's no shortage of unpleasant life-changing or life-destroying illnesses to choose from, if you've seen enough full-on depressive episodes, you would understand that depression is among the worse of them. I still vividly recall a conversation with a fellow psychiatrist who told me about one of his depressed patients. This man's depression was so severe that he had developed a delusional belief that his insides were rotting and that he might already be dead. He actually took himself to the cemetery and lay down there, waiting for someone to shovel earth over him. I can't imagine the state of mind of someone who does that, what despair and anguish leads to that point, but I do know that I would never want me or anyone I cared about to experience it.

In depression, patients experience a profound sense of misery, despair, and hopelessness. Feelings of regret, worthlessness, guilt, and shame become intolerable. The past is seen as a series of failures, the present as a period of pointless suffering, and the future as a slough of hopelessness and futility. This mood saturates all their interactions. (As a medical student I once saw a depressed woman on an inpatient ward, introduced myself, and asked if I could speak to her. She stared at the floor, waited a while, and then, oblivious to the well-justified debauched reputation of medical students, could only think to say, in a drab monotone, "It can't be much fun being a medical student.") Depressed people stop sleeping, stop eating, and become socially withdrawn and unable to work; thoughts of death and dying become persistent. Suicidal thoughts are never far away, and nearly always present, sometimes as a fantasy and means of escape and sometimes as a clear-cut and thought-through plan.

As I sat with Simon in my office, a sense of gloom and anguish seemed to fill the room. He just radiated these emotions. It was winter, but we were roasting hot. Outside, the sky was darkening, and inside, the fluorescent light hummed, the clock ticked, and my voice seemed to become quieter to match his, although in fact he spoke little and mostly looked down at the floor. His life was going down the tubes. He couldn't concentrate at work and had started to make mistakes. He wasn't sleeping, had stopped eating, and was losing weight. His clothes seemed to hang off him. He said that ordinary conversations had become an ordeal. Banter at work was exhausting. When someone cracked a joke, he could see the point of it but just didn't find it funny. He believed, against all evidence, that his past had been a failure. He saw minor disagreements as proof that he was a bad person and revisited in his mind long-forgotten events at school. He began to worry that he might have been a bully and hoped that those he tormented could see him suffering now, so they could see that he had received his just deserts. I found this so poignant and sad that I lost my way for a moment. I asked him if he thought things might get better in the future. He shook his head. He saw the future as bleak, a time over which he had no control, so what was the point in trying?

It brought to mind a study that I hadn't thought much about since medical school. This was an animal model for human depression. Animal models are an attempt to extrapolate, from animal data, the likely causes of illness in humans. In this experiment, there were two groups of dogs, beagles as I recall, each group sitting on a metal plate. A buzzer sounded and then an electric shock was applied to the plate. Nothing seriously harmful, but certainly unpleasant and enough to make the dogs want to get off the plate, which they could do by jumping over a little fence and onto the metal plate on the other side.

The first group of beagles had previously been conditioned to know that they could escape electric shocks if they tried. The second group of dogs had been previously conditioned to believe they had no control over electric shocks. So when the buzzer sounded, the first group of dogs quickly leaped over to the other side to escape the shock, but the second group of dogs didn't even try to escape, even though if they had, they would have discovered the experimenters had turned off the electric charge on the other side. The second group of dogs lay on the mildly charged floor, looking listless and dejected, whining, convinced that nothing they could do for themselves would improve their outcome. This image stuck in my mind: listless, depressed beagles, passive and accepting of their fate.

I'm not sure if an experiment like that would get ethical approval in this day and age, but it did tell us something important about learned helplessness in humans and its relationship to depression. The theory seems quite persuasive. Imagine that you've spent your whole life being told that everything is out of your reach, that no matter how hard you try, you'll never reach your goals. Success is something that happens only to other people. It must be tempting after a while just not to bother. It seems easier to simply give up when something is not working out, and this only reinforces the idea that nothing you do will ever work out. And once you stop trying, it won't be long before opportunities stop presenting themselves and life passes you by. In an awful, self-fulfilling way, learned helplessness leads to apathy and depression, and another life is lost in the hinterland of futility and despair.

So if life experiences account for depression, why then do we resort to talk about chemical transmitters in the brain when we try to explain to patients why they are depressed? Well, it seems that neurotransmitters are at least part of the explanation. Deficiencies of neurotransmitters such as serotonin, noradrenaline, and possibly dopamine appear to be important in the development of depression. Billions of neurons, synaptic connections, and neurotransmitters contribute to our personalities and the development of psychological problems. Depression is a result of our genetic predisposition, perhaps influencing the wiring of our brain and chemical transmitters. These in turn are influenced by our experiences, by our behavioral and coping styles, and by life events.

When I suggest antidepressants to patients, many look pretty nervous at the prospect, uneasy at taking something that could affect the function of their mind—although I note that people nearly always have a more relaxed attitude toward other things that may affect their mind, such as alcohol or cannabis. But I do understand the reluctance some people have toward antidepressants. I think I would feel equally nervous about having a hip replacement, but if you need one, you need one. And so I take a similarly pragmatic approach to treatment with antidepressants. Nobody really wants to be on them, but then nobody really wants to be ill in the first place. There's no doubt, though, that if anti-depressants are prescribed with care, they work and transform lives. They certainly did with Simon. When I saw him a few weeks later, there was the glimmer of something changing. He said he had been sleeping a little better, was less irritable, and was not quite as anxious. As the weeks passed, his mood gradually improved. I remember my surprise one day when he cracked a joke as he came into the clinic room from the waiting room. He told me that he was now back at work and things were going well. He had a sex life once more, he enjoyed being with his family, and they were relieved to have him back.

Depression can be one of the most satisfying illnesses to treat. Yet on a fairly regular basis the patient will show an unwillingness to take treatment, a reluctance that can be hard to counter, so that half the battle in successful treatment of depression can be in persuading the patient that they actually need treatment at all. There are some people for whom this response is an inherent part of their depression. I have seen patients so depressed that they believe that they are worthless or that they deserve to suffer. They tell me that they think my time would be better spent with someone else.

More commonly, though, the illness itself is not the problem. Instead it is the prejudice of the poorly informed or the misinformed, as well as the misleading information about the illness and its treatments widely available on the internet and in the press, that permeates the public consciousness and contributes to the general misunderstanding of the illness. Much has been written about the "pill shaming" of people who do choose to take antidepressant medication. This term refers to the criticism on social media directed toward people taking psychiatric treatment and seems to be exclusively aimed at medication for mental illness. I have seen it myself and shake my head in bewilderment at the hostility directed toward individuals who admit to being in treatment. I wonder what business it is of others to question someone's choice of how to treat their illness. You simply don't get that level of antipathy toward treatment for physical illness; no one criticizes a person's choice to have a cardiac bypass, for example. But mental illness is a special case, touching as it does on the essence of our very being, and maybe the attitudes toward the treatment are simply a reflection of that fear.

ALTRUISM

I wonder if many of us think about our legacy of our time on earth. If we do, what sort of legacy will it be? How do we want to be remembered? I think most of us, given opportunities to do a kindness to a fellow human, would do so. Most of these will be through small acts—say, a charitable donation or help given to a stranger—and of course would not intersect with healthcare at all. Yet in some cases the altruistic act turns individuals into patients, moving them into the healthcare system and from there into the clinic of a psychiatrist.

What would it take for you to give away one of your kidneys? To voluntarily become a patient, entangled in the hospital system, when you didn't really have to be there at all? I suppose if the situation demanded it, you might give a kidney to a close relative—a child, say, a sibling, or perhaps a parent. A close friend, at a stretch. When I was first appointed as a consultant psychiatrist in 2003, working in a large London teaching hospital with an active transplant program, kidney donation consisted almost entirely of a parent giving their kidney to a child or sometimes a sibling. Giving your kidney to the hospital without specifying at all who was to get it—that is, giving it to a stranger whom you would never get to meet—was something that Americans did, it being legal in the United States some time before it became legal in the UK.

Nearly everyone is born with two kidneys. People who are born with one kidney usually never find this out, because they feel perfectly healthy, and sometimes the first time they discover they have only one kidney is when they offer to be a donor. The function of kidneys is to filter waste products from the blood and to regulate fluid levels in the body. Without functioning kidneys, toxins build up, and these make people feel progressively unwell. And without normal kidneys, people do not produce urine, and fluid overload can make them swell up, making it hard to breathe. Dialysis machines can replicate the function of a kidney, but unlike a dialysis machine, a real kidney is always working. Patients on dialysis need to come to the hospital three times a week to be connected to a dialysis machine for four hours at a time. Blood is taken out of the body, filtered by the machine, and returned to the body, cleansed. Many patients describe the experience as draining, and life becomes a never-ending cycle of dialysis and recovery. A life on dialysis can be very restrictive, not just because of the obvious things like the time spent doing it, which involves long swaths of boredom. But additionally, dialysis eats into patients' working lives and vacations. For most patients I see, the vacation issue is usually resolved by not going on holiday at all.

Kidney transplants are a solution that offers a degree of freedom to patients and are usually the goal toward which dialysis patients strive. Kidney transplants are not an easy option. Aside from an operation, a transplant involves taking anti-rejection medication every day to stop the body from rejecting the new kidney, and of course the medication comes with side effects. But if it works well, a transplant offers a great deal more freedom than being on dialysis, and life can get back to something approaching normal, which is why this option is preferred by most people if it's available. The problem is that commonly it's not. Spare kidneys are hard to come by, with approximately 5,000 people currently waiting on the transplant list in the UK. In the United States, the average wait time for a kidney to become available is in the order of four years.

Most kidneys for transplant come from people who have died and who have requested that their organs be donated after death. Not all of those kidneys will be of high quality. They can vary depending on the age of the person at death and the circumstances surrounding their death. So, for example, a young person dying tragically in a motorcycle accident is likely to have a kidney in better shape to donate than one from someone older who has died of a serious disease. A second consideration is the period of time that elapses between the donor's dying and a match being found, as well as the time involved in getting the kidney to them (it could be at the other end of the country). As you might expect, the greater the delay, the worse the outcome. Finally, kidneys need to be matched to the recipient, and strangers can be harder to match than a closer relative. Our bodies are designed to get rid of anything that looks alien to them, which is usually a good thing when you are fighting off an infection, but the body also notices the myriad differences between its own kidney and a transplanted one. Once the body notices differences in a transplanted kidney, it will try to fight it off, a process known as rejection. So the closer the match between the donor and recipient—taking into account all the hundreds of markers by which a body can tell friend from foe—the better the outcome.

To make up the shortfall in kidneys, the practice of living donation (which happens while the donor is still alive) has been steadily increasing over the years. Approximately a third of donations are now from a living donor. Yet this brings with it a new ethical question. If the kidney donor is not improved physically by undergoing an operation—indeed, is sometimes even worse off physically after giving a kidney away—then this is the exact opposite of what we are normally trying to achieve in medicine. So what, then, is our justification for taking a kidney from someone? If the donor does not benefit physically, any benefits have to be psychological—for example, the pleasure gained from a selfless act— or at the very least not lead to psychological harm. It was for this reason that psychiatrists first became involved in the whole area of kidney donations. They were needed to make a judgment as to whether some- one was psychologically robust enough to undergo the operation, particularly in the early days of transplants, when the success of the operation was far from guaranteed.

Kidney transplants have been around since the 1960s, although they were less common and riskier operations then. Patient selection, for both donor and recipient, was more careful, because of the relative rar- ity of the operation. In the early years of transplants, concerns were raised about possible coercion of the donor and the psychological risks of donating. Imagine the following scenario: You are sitting in your boss's office, having a cup of tea and discussing whatever people talk about with their boss. At the end of the discussion, as you pause and ask if there is anything else, the boss indicates that there is, so you settle back down into your seat. Your boss appears to choose her words care- fully, saying that she has come to consider you, over the past couple of years, as a friend. In that spirit, she goes on to say, for a while now she has needed a kidney. She talks to you about the difficulties of life on dialysis, the perpetual exhaustion, discomfort, itching, boredom, all of which would be made so much better with a transplant. She would like you to consider whether you might possibly consider coming forward as a kidney donor. No pressure, she hastens to add: no, just something to think about. And please, of course, don't worry, you can forget the conversation ever happened if you want.

Now, how would you feel? No actual pressure has been brought to bear, no expectation of anything, just what may seem like a reasonable and sensitively communicated request. Yet now that the subject has been raised, you find yourself in a difficult situation. The possibility is in the air between you and your boss every time you see each other. And because of the disparity in your respective positions, you may end up feeling a pressure to say yes to something that you very much do not want to do, or say no and sense the boss's daily disappointment at, and for all you know resentment of, your decision.

Similarly, in families where the power dynamics are unequal, feelings of coercion are not uncommon. I have seen this scenario on several occasions. I recall seeing Alana, a woman in her twenties who had come forward to offer a kidney to her father. All of her siblings had offered to donate a kidney for their father, but it turned out that Alana was the closest match. A little way into the consultation, I asked about her relationship with her father, a fairly standard sort of question to ask of someone considering donating. Her reply was correct, but in a formulaic and mechanical sort of way. Everything she said, written on paper, would make her appear to be an ideal donor. Yes, she loved her father, was concerned for his health, and wanted to donate a kidney. Yet there was something about the way she spoke, rather than what she said, that made me sit up. Her answers lacked any emotional warmth, being correct rather than sincere, and I began to form the impression that despite her words, she disliked her father.

I put it to her that there seemed to be more that she wasn't saying. She asked, as patients sometimes do before deciding to say something more significant, whether this interview was confidential. She hesitantly began her story, although she appeared worried. She was fearful of being blamed for "failing" the psychiatric assessment, although she seemed keen to talk, if she could dissociate herself from the consequences. She began to talk about her childhood. She was the child who was sent to a state school because she was not academically talented, while two of her other siblings were given a private education, with all the advantages that conferred. This history itself was irksome to her, as she struggled to understand how a father could treat his children so differently, but what she really resented was her father's favoritism toward her more academic siblings. This came out in ways big and small, such as allowing her siblings to go to the Model United Nations with their school, but not allowing her to go on a holiday with her friends to compensate. It seemed to her that her father always sat her siblings nearer to him at dinner, sought their advice, laughed at their jokes, and admired their careers. It was difficult to tell how much of this was reality and how much was a story she had constructed for herself, and which she now saw everywhere because she was always on the lookout for evidence. Either way, years of frustration, disappointment, and resentment had built up. It seemed to me that donating a kidney was something she really did not want to do, although she was prepared to go through with it, rather than to say how she felt directly.

I waited for the right moment, although I felt uneasy. As we discussed the pros and cons of the operation, I directed the discussion as to whether she would feel able to back out of the proposed donation should she change her mind. There was a pause. I asked the question again, although I phrased it differently: "How would you feel if the hospital found a reason to disqualify you from donating a kidney?" There was another pause. Then I added: "Would it be a disappointment . . . or perhaps a relief?"

At that moment, I was presented with another of those scenes that you see on dramas but rarely in real life. Her shoulders slumped dramatically, all the tension now gone, so that she looked like a puppet when the strings have been cut, her head dropped to her chest. She exhaled shakily. Tears started to well up in her eyes. The relief was evident, even as she tried to conceal her delight that someone had finally picked up that she was going through the motions only to please her family. She just wanted someone to notice and to stop her so that she could be absolved of any blame. I wondered now about her father, desperately hoping for a kidney to change his life, giving him freedom from dialysis. My responsibilities were to the patient in front of me, and her father was not my patient, but I wasn't sure then, and I'm still not sure now, to what extent this was a good outcome.

It was one of those consultations that was all about the mood, the nuance—how things were said rather than what was being said. It is what the psychotherapists sometimes call "listening with your third ear," when you hear what is not being said rather than simply focusing on the words, because beneath the words there is a whole different communication going on. If I had not been paying attention or if I had accepted at face value what I was being told, I would have nodded through what would on the surface have appeared to be an entirely reasonable and understandable wish to donate. Alana would have given away a kidney and resented every moment of it. Such are the psychological pressures when the idea of kidney donation is even raised. I understood why a commentator in one of the journals dubbed a request for kidney donation a "call to self-sacrifice." I think this is probably an exaggeration, but I got the point.

Things are often fraught when the donor and the recipient know each other. Sometimes the donor comes forward because they are secretly hoping for a change in relationship with the recipient, a lasting gratitude that will forever bind them together. The recipient, by contrast, may simply want a kidney so that he or she can come off dialysis and start a new life, and the donor is simply a means to that end. In my experience, any ambiguity in the relationship between recipient and donor can spell disaster. A kidney needs to be a gift given unconditionally. There can be no strings attached, no "Where do you think you're going with my kidney at this time of night?"

My experience, though, is that the majority of donors do not regret the decision to donate. In fact, most people say that they would make the same choice if they were given it again. When asked, people say that the act of donation improved their self-esteem and gave them a renewed sense of purpose in life. For these people, giving a kidney away can actually improve their health rather than worsen it, and improved self-esteem can lead to benefits in all aspects of an individual's life, including relationships, friendships, and work life.

As kidney transplants have become more routine, attitudes have eased. Donors are no longer being told that donating their kidney to a relative is a trap, involving some kind of coercion. Instead, the opposite problem has developed. These are the psychological effects of denying someone the opportunity to donate and making them stand helplessly aside while their loved one suffers the ongoing grind of dialysis. Sometimes I am faced with the question as to which is the greater risk to a patient's mental health and well-being. Is it the risk of donating or of not donating? Over the course of my career, there has undoubtedly been a shift in societal values informing decisions like this. The balance of decision-making has changed: the patient's opinion is the most heavily weighted factor out of all the considerations. The era of "doctor knows best" is now anathema, and medical paternalism seems to encapsulate what people imagine to be the very worst of medical practice.

I have regularly been involved in assessing donors when they have had a past psychiatric history. This raises the question as to whether the stress of giving a kidney, particularly if things don't run smoothly, risks reactivating the psychiatric problem and making everything worse. The problem I face is of the patients' understanding of risk and their attitude toward it. Not exactly psychiatry, but not entirely unconnected with it, either. *Thinking, Fast and Slow* by Daniel Kahneman is a marvelous book that sets out how people think about risk and how emotion and gut feelings, rather than rationality, influence how individuals behave. This applies to people of all levels of education. Kahneman shows how people have an intuitive understanding of risk that is often quite at odds with the reality. For example, an individual's perception of risk may change according to how worthwhile they think the operation is. If they see kidney donation as pointless, adding little to the quality of a recipient's life, they are more likely to see the operation as risky and dangerous. And conversely, if they see an operation as a wonderful opportunity to help someone they love, they are more likely to see the risks of the operation as much lower.

One of my favorite studies about how emotion overcomes reason was in a 1994 paper by Veronica Denes-Raj and Seymour Epstein. Subjects were told that they would win $1 for each time they picked a red jelly bean out of a covered jar. One jar (A) had nine white jelly beans and one red, so it offered a 1 in 10 chance of picking out the red jelly bean. Another jar (B) had a hundred jelly beans, ninety-one white and nine red, so there was a 9 in 100 chance of picking out a red jelly bean. Which jar would you pick?

Well, logically it has to be jar A, because there is a 1 in 10 chance from jar A, but only a 9 in 100 chance (which is less than 1 in 10) of picking the red jelly bean from jar B. Yet a majority of subjects (61 percent) picked jar B. The question is, why would people make a choice that they know is the wrong one? Well, the answer is that it is an emotional choice. Subjects knew they were making the wrong choice from a mathematical point of view, yet emotionally they just felt that there was a greater chance of picking a red jelly bean if there were more of them, which is why jar B was so tempting. It is a choice that literally defies logic, yet people make decisions like this all the time. When it comes to these kinds of decisions in healthcare, the same thinking patterns are replicated. But if doctors think, for example, that where kidney donation is concerned, the patient is not seeing the risks clearly, to what extent should they step in, and to what extent should they respect patient autonomy?

I remember seeing Robert, a man in his thirties, who had been asked by his sister's husband if he would consider giving a kidney to his sister. She had been on dialysis for years, although Robert wasn't too sure what had happened to make her kidneys fail. He thought perhaps a childhood illness had damaged them. He had a recollection when they were children of her being in the hospital. He remembered her face being quite puffy but couldn't remember any other details of her hospital stay, only that he had to stay with his grandparents for a week.

They grew up in the Lake District, in a small semidetached house. His father worked in one of the national parks, maintaining footpaths and bridges, and his mother worked as a receptionist in a nearby hotel. He recalled his childhood as a happy one. He and his sister weren't particularly close, though. There was an age gap of only two years between them, and there were no other siblings in the family, yet they did not share the confidences that siblings often do, did not play together when they were growing up, and didn't mix in the same social circles as teenagers.

Robert told me that he left school at the first opportunity and worked in the hospitality industry for a couple of years. Then he moved to London, where he had his first manic episode, although his recollection of it was a little hazy. (After the appointment, I got the old notes from the hospital where he had been admitted with his manic episode. It was worse than he had remembered it. He had tried to buy a boat, even though he had never sailed, with the intention of sailing around the world. The exuberance and overconfidence of his manic episode had caused him to disregard any objections, and it seems the purchase went through.) His euphoria had quickly given way to irritability over the subsequent days. He became frustrated to the point of exasperation with people who were unable to keep up with his racing thoughts and his pressured speech. Soon, though, irritability gave way to a deep depression, as his mania started to resolve with the treatment he had been given, and he began to reflect on the enormity of what had happened. He had lost a great deal of money buying a secondhand boat at an inflated price, he had jeopardized his relationships, but most of all, he feared for what the future might hold.

The fear was justified. He had three relapses over the next few years, on one occasion being admitted to a hospital for five weeks. Outside of his episodes, though, his life was progressing. He found a job working for the local council as a gardener. He married in his mid-twenties and had two children. Unfortunately, during one of his manic episodes a few years later, he spent a substantial amount of his savings on another harebrained scheme, a landscaping project that had no hope of being commissioned, and in despair and exasperation, his wife left him. He told me about this time in his life, when he thought that he would lose everything. He found that the psychological pain in the aftermath of an episode was worse than anything he had experienced, and much worse than the manic episodes, which he actually found quite enjoyable. He told me that he loved the euphoria that came with the mania—his boundless enthusiasm, the energy, and the feeling that anything was possible and that the world would bend to his will. The lows that followed, though, were a special form of torment for him. These were not clear-cut depressive episodes, but rather a form of reckoning. They were a debt that now needed to be paid off, where all the things he had done and said, all the money he had spent, all the indiscreet sexual liaisons that had happened in the throes of his mania when he felt indomitable, now had to be accounted for. All the remorse and shame and guilt, the recriminations and tears and anger—these were the things that caused him the most pain and suffering.

I looked at Robert sitting across the desk from me. "You realize that the stress of the operation may be a trigger for a relapse of your bipolar illness? Particularly if things don't run smoothly." My experience has been that people say that they understand the risks of the transplant operation, of pain, of bleeding, of infections—even the risk of operative deaths, which happens with a frequency of about 1 in 3,000. But nearly all the patients I see think that the risk applies to other people, not to them. "There's also the risk that the kidney might not work, and through nobody's fault, all this might have been for nothing." Robert nodded, and there was silence. He sat opposite me in a pair of outdoor trousers and a fleece that had seen better days, his sturdy pair of boots tapping with agitation under the desk. "Are you sure about this?" I asked. "After all, you're not particularly close to your sister."

He thought about his response. "I come from a small family. I didn't grow up with uncles and aunts fussing over me. My sister is the only real relative I've got, and anyway I gave her my word."

"But what if the operation, the hospital stay, perhaps the complications of an operation are enough to trigger another bipolar episode?"

"Well, that could happen anytime, couldn't it?" And of course this was true: a bipolar episode could happen at any time, and it was difficult to quantify the extra risk of the operation. I was pretty sure the risk was likely to be increased, though, particularly if things went wrong and his brief hospital stay became a longer affair accompanied by pain, infection, and sleepless nights—but it was difficult to say by how much the risk would be increased.

How people think about risk is also affected by how you ask the question, something known as framing. As Kahneman shows, if you ask subjects the same question but phrase it differently, then you get very different answers. Again, an individual's approach to risk can be affected by factors that really shouldn't matter. In one study, colleagues of mine at Guy's Hospital asked potential kidney donors what risk they would accept as a kidney donor. They showed that what is already known to be true in other contexts is also true of kidney donors. Where risk is presented as "chance of survival" rather than "risk of death," donors are more likely to accept a higher risk, particularly for a close relative who is unwell. So a 90 percent chance of survival is seen much more favorably than a 10 percent risk of death, even though these are the same thing.

However, that was not the most surprising discovery in the paper. What jumped out at me was how risky an operation would have to be for a potential donor to consider the risk too high. While the accepted figure of operative death for a kidney donor is about 1 in 3,000, the most common figure that potential donors would find an acceptable risk was 1 in 2! In other words, a fifty-fifty chance of coming through the operation, which 29 percent of the donors said they would accept. This leads back to the discussions about paternalism and medical practice. I don't think any doctor would subject a healthy volunteer to a 50 percent chance of death to save a relative. And I suspect that patients would expect doctors to refuse to operate if the risk was too high, to manage risk for them in much the same way that I don't expect to be consulted by someone piloting a plane I am on about weather conditions and whether he should fly, even if I desperately want to reach the destination. On the other hand, whose risk is it to take, for an adult with capacity to make decisions?

When I asked this question with respect to Robert during a lecture at a national kidney conference, before an audience of kidney doctors, nurses, transplant surgeons, and psychologists, the room was divided almost exactly fifty-fifty about whether they thought Robert should donate or not be allowed to. The dilemma I put to them was that this was an unquantifiable but likely increased risk of a relapse of bipolar disorder, knowing that previous relapses had caused significant emotional and psychological harm. Added to this are all the self-serving biases, in which people who are taking risks under conditions of uncertainty tend to see what they want to see, to support their decision rather than to challenge it. If you were deciding, what would you have done? Would you have recommended he be allowed to make the donation?

At the clinic appointment with Robert, I struggled with my decision. Was my responsibility to protect Robert from himself? Or was it to accept that if he seemed to understand the risks, even if he didn't really think they would apply to him, that would be enough? I eventually went with the latter view, and Robert went ahead and had the operation three months after I saw him. Despite a few nervous moments three days postoperatively, when he seemed to be a bit more energetic and overfamiliar, a few good nights of sleep seemed to straighten him out, and six months later he had not had the manic episode I had feared. In fact, he said that he felt much better about himself, and that this was one good thing in his life he could feel proud of, despite everything else that had happened to him.

Robert was on my mind some months later as I sat in my office, with the view of the futuristic Shard skyscraper through the window. I was wondering what to do about a new case, this time an altruistic donor named Luke, whom I had seen that morning. Altruistic donations are those in which donors choose to give a kidney to whoever needs one, someone they don't know and whom in all likelihood they will never get to meet.

My early interactions with altruistic donors were characterized by an uncertainty bordering on mistrust of their motives. At the very least, I felt they had to present their case to a psychiatrist. Since they were not benefiting physically from their donation in any way and they had no connection to the recipient, then why on earth were they doing this? Where was the gain? What possible reason would someone have for donating a kidney to a stranger who might never even thank them? How would you know the surgeon hadn't dropped your kidney by mistake on the operating room floor? There was little UK guidance on assessments of altruistic donors, although I was able to reference some studies in the United States and set to work gaining my own database of donors, to offer some basis for what would soon become a very interesting source of work, with centers from London and the southeast of England referring potential altruistic kidney donors to me.

My experience of altruistic kidney donors has been that their motives vary widely, and they defy attempts to pigeonhole them into any particular category. I would say that the only common theme among them is that they want to do something remarkable and selfless, and it is their wish to do it in an extreme way that sets them aside from the rest of the population. Sometimes the reason seems understandable—for example, they have known people who have benefited from NHS care or from having received a kidney, or they have a particular connection or sympathy with the plight of patients on dialysis. Other times there is an underpinning philosophy, a desire to change the world. I have heard patients say that the distribution of wealth, power, and privilege is so uneven, so unprincipled, that they want to try to level things out as best they can. To them, giving a kidney is a step toward their goal. Often they will have been charity volunteers or work in the charity sector, but not all of them. Some work in finance, some in local government, others in healthcare—all types of profession are represented. The youngest donor I have assessed was eighteen, and the oldest were in their seventies. I have seen workers who earn modestly give at least 10 percent of their income to charity, and some have been so inspirational that at one point I began to consider if I should donate a kidney.

By contrast, some patients who want to donate are unencumbered by lofty philosophical principles. In a recent consultation, a young man in his early thirties told me that he had seen something about donation on the television and decided that he should do that. He explained that "I've always known you don't need both of them [his kidneys] . . .

I've got no strong reason not to." I told him that many people were in exactly his position and would find plenty of strong reasons not to, but he just shrugged and said, "You help people out where you can." I kept returning to the theme of motivation, trying to find some deep-seated reason why he was doing this, but it turned out that for him, it really was as simple as that. He just didn't see giving a kidney as a big deal; he didn't think it should be.

There are other reasons to give a kidney that can feel a little more on the borderline. Some potential donors are lonely. They want to feel that the physicians and surgeons are their professional colleagues and friends, rather than clinicians who have a dispassionate and professional interest in their care. The motivation is to fill a void in their lives, the gap friendships and families normally fill. I've come up against this a few times, and my experience has taught me that this does not always end well. The answer to a lack of companionship is not to try to make the professionals caring for you into friends.

I have seen individuals come forward as donors for whom the act of giving a kidney was more akin to an act of self-harm than an altruistic act, only self-harm inflicted by the hospital. It's the medical equivalent of what is often called "suicide by cop." I recall seeing one patient and finding it difficult to discern his motives for the kidney donation, but nothing really alarmed me, either. I assumed he was just someone who was not given to much self-reflection, someone who wanted to act rather than think about the significance of the act. I wondered whether he should proceed with the donation process and came to the conclusion that I couldn't really see why not—that is, until I received a phone call from one of the transplant nurses, who alerted me to the medical notes from another hospital. I had no idea why they weren't sent to me. I hadn't even realized they existed. It made for grim reading. As I flicked through a photocopy of the notes when they arrived a few days later, I read with growing alarm about a recent hospital admission after the patient had swallowed button batteries (a surprisingly dangerous thing to do). There were numerous episodes in casualty following overdoses. I had missed all of this when I spoke to him, or rather he withheld it from me, and for some reason it wasn't on the GP records that I'd requested. The whole situation had me rattled. I asked to see him again, which I did a couple of weeks later. I told him of the notes from the other hospital that I had now seen and asked why he hadn't told me any of this when I'd asked specifically about his past medical and psychiatric history and any previous instances of self-harm. He told me he didn't think it was relevant. I wonder if he had asked his GP to withhold that information from me, too, as I couldn't think of any other reason that I wouldn't have been told about it. I considered what would have happened if he had proceeded to surgery, but since I declined to support the procedure, this question remained unanswered.

Usually I am able to make up my mind about the psychological suitability of someone to give a kidney to the hospital, but there are times when I find myself uncertain of what constitutes a reasonable and acceptable motive, a question that goes to the heart of what altruism is, and whether there is such a thing as pure altruism. I remember seeing Luke in my outpatient clinic one spring afternoon. He was in his mid-thirties, and through the downstairs window in my clinic room, the one with the internal view into the hospital, I saw him wheel his bike, with what looked like snow on the frame, half wheeling it along and then jumping on it for a bit like a teenager on a skateboard, as he made his way to the corridor where my clinic was taking place. Although I didn't know at the time that he would eventually be my patient, as I watched him pass by my window, I idly thought that he was the inverse of me. I looked at myself—gray suit, white shirt, dark blue tie, black brogues, and a neatly clipped head, not quite shaved, but the modern bald look.

I put myself in the category of basically kind, but I probably take myself too seriously. Sharp sense of humor, lying dormant, suffocated under layers of roles and responsibilities.

Luke, by contrast, was all bonhomie. He wore jeans, sandals, and a collarless hemp shirt, with his sleeves rolled up to his elbows to reveal almost hairless arms and a variety of string bracelets. He had a thicket of matte brown hair, shoulder length and uncombed, and guileless gray-blue eyes. As he entered my office, I glanced back at the referral letter, which said that he had come forward as an altruistic kidney donor. We exchanged small talk (he had cycled three miles to the appointment, and cycling was his favorite mode of transport) before getting to why he had come to see me. He wanted to give his kidney away "because when I die, I want to be able to die knowing I did one good thing."

He told me he had grown up in an affluent part of England and had gone to an expensive private school about a forty-minute drive from his house. His father, a self-made man, commuted each day into the center of London, where he ran a large property company. His father had started the company from scratch before he married, and he never tired of telling the family how he had pulled himself up from nothing, and that all it took was dedication and hard work.

Luke said that he was easily influenced at school and had little respect for authority, so he regularly found himself in trouble. At first this was for answering back to teachers and disrupting classes. Soon, though, he began to skip school so that he could fit in with his friends, but inevitably he was caught. Despite his behavioral problems, he was a bright young man, yet the school had clearly had enough of him and he was eventually expelled. As he was sixteen, he was allowed to take his GCSE exams, the set of national exams taken by almost everyone in the UK at that age, but by then he had given up on his education and failed most of them.

His father was furious. All that expensive education, he said, and this was how he was repaid. He decided that Luke would go to work, get a taste of the real world, understand the value of hard labor and the value of money. He was given a low-paying entry-level job in property, to show him the business from the bottom up. Luke, though, saw this as punitive, a humiliation. His friends laughed at him, and he tried to laugh along, but he was outraged by what had happened and believed that he didn't deserve to be treated like this. He began to supplement his income by selling cannabis to friends.

Over time his drug-selling operation grew, and his interest in property waned. He began to deal in bigger quantities of drugs and had an aptitude for the business. He told me that it was the first thing he had done that he excelled at. His father suspected what was going on and threw him out of the house.

He continued his dealing, and over the next few years began a relationship, had a child, and lived together with his partner and daughter until his past caught up with him. He was arrested in the early hours one morning at his flat, and after a trial was sentenced to six years in prison. During this time, his partner left him. At this point his voice cracked and his chin trembled with the effort not to cry, and it was a few moments before he continued. He did not see his daughter for several years after this, and initially did not even know where she was. His partner considered him a bad influence, said she wanted nothing more to do with him, and married just before his release from prison.

"After that I just fell apart," he told me, his eyes red, rubbing them with a tissue. He was by now in his late twenties; he had no qualifications, a prison record, and no relationship, and his family had all but disowned him. He thought of suicide and on one occasion took too many tablets, although he never seriously thought that would work, and on reflection said it was a mixture of desperation and self-pity, not any real wish to be dead.

His life never really got back on track. He worked at a series of menial part-time jobs, but he did not build a career and had no stable social life. He had short-term relationships but nothing that lasted more than a few months, and so his life drifted by. He told me that he had "never done one good thing" with his life, so when he heard about the possibility of organ donation, he realized that this could be it. Whatever the shortcomings of his life to that point, if he gave a kidney, he could die knowing that there was one incontrovertible act of good that he had committed in this world.

Psychiatry has taught me a lot of things, but this was not about mental illness, it was about making a judgment on someone's life and motives, was about whether there is truly such a thing as altruism. I have heard the old argument that there's no such thing as a free lunch, that there is always some aspect of selfishness in every altruistic act. Maybe there is, but we can never know, and I can't see why that would change anything even if it was true. Perhaps all donors are the same as Luke to a greater or lesser degree, hoping to fulfill some need deep within themselves. I wondered in Luke's case whether it made sense to allow someone to expiate guilt through an act of donation. And would it in fact finally give him some peace of mind, some compensation for all those wasted years? I was doubtful. The things we believe will make our lives complete tend to give only transient satisfaction. The commonly held notion that money will resolve all our cares and lead to happiness is a fallacy, as studies of lottery winners have shown. But the promise of happiness gained from money and the happiness resulting from the deeper satisfaction of an altruistic act are very different. And after all, who am I to decide what will give someone's life meaning or bring happiness? In the end I didn't raise any objections to Luke donating, and I hope he found the peace of mind that he was looking for.

EXHAUSTION

When I first saw Carole, she was asleep on a small purple sofa in the waiting room. We had recently put the sofa there, at the suggestion of the local ME support group. ME is short for myalgic encephalomyelitis, the name given to a controversial illness commonly called chronic fatigue syndrome (CFS), an illness that I have specialized in over the past twenty years. The ME group thought a sofa would be helpful for our patients, and it certainly was for Carole. Looking at her, I realized that she had not just dozed off but was lying with her head flopped backward, her mouth open, as if she had been anesthetized. I entered the waiting room and called her name, and she barely stirred. I bent down and spoke her name directly into her ear, and this time there was a groggy opening of the eyes, then a look that was somewhere between startled and bewildered. She slowly maneuvered around until her feet were touching the floor, took a moment as she seemed to will herself to stand upright, then got to her feet and followed me down the long corridor, past the small wilted cactus on the window ledge, and through two sets of fire doors before finally arriving at my office.

The referral letter from her GP included clinical notes from her repeated visits to him over the past few years, with "TATT" written at the beginning of most entries. Doctors use such acronyms less and less, relics of a bygone era, because some of them were rather uncomplimentary to the patient, although the relatively benign TATT stood for "tired all the time." Carole was thirty-eight at this point and told me she had had symptoms exactly half her life, first developing them at age nineteen while she was at university, after a bout of glandular fever. Initially she was laid low for a couple of weeks and took to her bed, confident that she would soon be back on her feet. She was in a hurry to recover, and thus before she was fully well, she tried to catch up with some of the course work that she had missed, aware that she was starting to fall behind. She recalled that the stress of this made her worse, and she began to spiral downward. By the end of the second term she was spending twelve hours of the day in bed, yet still felt unrefreshed when she woke in the morning. Her muscles ached. She developed headaches and sore throats. She was exhausted all the time, and even minimal exertion such as running for a bus would leave her bed-bound for days afterward. Her biggest problems were the cognitive symptoms of poor concentration and worsening short-term memory. This meant that studying was far more difficult, her exam performance suffered, and her expected progression into the workplace and beyond never materialized.

Carole told me she was single and still lived at home in her parents' house. She had managed little more than part-time work, but with an unreliable employment record, she found it difficult to advance in the workplace or even to hold down a job. Her parents had to cook for her, and she had been able to contribute little to the household. By the time she came to see me, she was in despair. She told me that it had been an uphill struggle to convince people, including her GP, that she was ill. She was aware of skepticism about her diagnosis among her family, her friends, and even her doctors, a skepticism that was often the worse for

being unspoken. She believed people saw her as lazy, flawed, even piti-
able, and told me what many patients in my fatigue clinic say to me—
that she sometimes wished she had a serious illness, because at least then
everyone would believe that she was suffering.

Feeling rejected by the medical profession, she undertook her own
research and consulted a number of nonmedical practitioners, many of
whom would deliver their own simplistic and medically fanciful theories about the illness, after which they would sell her their remedies. She
upended her bag of pills and supplements onto the desk. I counted
fourteen in total. These included berries, enzymes, supplements, miner-
als, vitamins, probiotics, and oxidant tablets as well as antioxidant tablets, the latter two a paradox that I didn't have the heart to point out to
her. All of these came at a princely sum that she had to borrow each
month from her parents. She told me that she felt driven to do this
because she wasn't getting any help from the medical profession.

This response is typical in my experience. Medicine's inability to
deal with a presentation that does not neatly fit into a diagnosis is something that has never been resolved, and people understandably seek
solutions elsewhere. Doctors deal in diagnoses, and so are always looking for the patterns in symptoms or investigation findings that will
confirm a particular diagnosis. Nearly all of our treatments are directed
at a diagnosis, rather than at the symptoms. So, for example, we have
treatments for angina, but not for chest pain, and treatments for rheu-
matoid arthritis but not for joint pain. For an individual presenting
with persistent exhaustion, if the doctor can't find a diagnosis to fit the
exhaustion, if exhaustion is a stand-alone symptom, then there is rarely
a proper treatment available. Doctors are uneasy about prescribing
treatments for symptoms, worrying that either they have missed the
proper diagnosis or they are providing non-evidence-based treatments.
Carole believed that her symptoms were dismissed by her doctors as
imagined, an impediment to their work of real disease, and her refusal

to get better was seen as deliberate and willful. Carole's suspicions seemed plausible. Negative attitudes toward CFS/ME are still fairly prevalent. The frustration of some doctors in dealing with presentations like Carole's, with hard-to-categorize illnesses that persist for years, is all too common.

My interest in chronic fatigue syndrome began when I was a junior doctor in internal medicine. What was this illness I kept reading about? Was it even real? I think I shared the same doubt about the diagnosis as most members of the public, and perhaps the same prejudices. What were we meant to call it, anyway? Some people use the term myalgic encephalomyelitis, which evokes an inflammation of the brain and spinal cord that has not been accepted by the medical profession. Doctors call it chronic fatigue syndrome, which many patients do not feel captures the full extent of their suffering. Sometimes the term "post-viral fatigue syndrome" has been used, but there are many others, and the lack of a consistent name is probably a reflection of the uncertainties, prejudices, or dogmas concerning the diagnosis. In some countries, doctors still refer to the illness as neurasthenia, a term whose origins go back to the nineteenth century in the United States, when it was described by the American neurologist George M. Beard. Beard ascribed the origins of the illness to the hectic pace of modern life, what with all those horses and buggies and telegrams to send.

I arrived at the Maudsley Hospital as a psychiatry trainee in 1996. The Maudsley is a famous old hospital in England, named after Henry Maudsley, the nineteenth-century British psychiatrist who founded the hospital. It was joined with the Bethlem Hospital a few miles away, to be known as the Bethlem and Maudsley. The Bethlem was even older, dating back to the thirteenth century (and its name is the origin of the word "bedlam," to describe a scene of chaos). Being accepted into their psychiatry training program was a proud moment, and I still clearly remember the euphoria of leaving internal medicine behind. Walking back to the car park on that warm spring evening after my first day in the job, I glanced over the road at King's College Hospital, the "medical" side of the road, and felt a rush of euphoria. No more would I have to do those brutal on-calls in internal medicine where I wouldn't return home for days on end, the never-ending clinics, the endless bleeps and pagers, the mountain of discharge letters, the breathless turnover of patients, the tyranny of endless guidelines—all these things were confined to a different time of my life. At least that was how it seemed then. But love is blind, and I had fallen in love with my new career, and the first day at least matched those expectations.

Throughout that long hot summer of 1996 I luxuriated in my new and far more interesting life in psychiatry. My journeys to work skipped along to the Lightning Seeds' unofficial anthem to the Euro 96 football tournament "Football's Coming Home," and England's serene progress to the semifinals of the tournament echoed my mood of optimism. I was at Wembley for England's unconvincing win over Spain in the quarterfinals, and back at the stadium days later to see the inevitable defeat to Germany in the semifinals. (I was reminded of the well-known quote from the famous England footballer Gary Lineker: "Football is a simple game. Twenty-two men chase a ball for ninety minutes, and in the end the Germans always win.") Yet even the cavorting German fans at the far end of the pitch, who had the gall to sing "Football's Coming Home" at the end of the match, didn't dampen my spirits too badly. I was working in my first job in psychiatry, in a locked intensive care ward, and seeing a whole new world of severe psychotic illness, including paranoid schizophrenia and bipolar disorder. I felt comfortable in the environment, a round peg in a round hole, and talked to patients about their auditory hallucinations, their delusional beliefs and paranoias, with a genuine fascination for the scale of the human experience.

My curiosity about chronic fatigue remained, though, and soon I got in contact with the hospital's specialist Chronic Fatigue Treatment and Research Unit, which years later was to become such a significant part of my working life. It was there that I met the person who has had the single biggest impact on my career, Dr. (and later Professor, and a little later still, Professor Sir) Simon Wessely. Simon is an extraordinary man. My first impression was that he looked like a cross between Art Garfunkel and John McEnroe. His shirt was tucked in at the front but not at the back; he wore dark blue chinos and no tie or jacket. He looked like what a man on the street would think a professor would look like, and in keeping with this, it did not take long for me to work out he was a genius. The first sign was his ability to get to the point of a problem and understand it more quickly than anyone I've met. His writing style is exactly the same as the way he talks—casual and informal, conversational, but touched by a sharp analysis of the problems. This applies to clinic letters, academic papers, conference talks, and, amazingly, policy documents. From my experience of being bored rigid by lengthy, dull, repetitive, derivative, and confused policy documents, I can say that the ability to make them seem interesting and relevant is so unusual as to be entirely unique.

At the time when Professor Wessely set up the chronic fatigue service, there was nothing similar available, and so waiting times for a first appointment were commonly two years. This led to an interesting fact. During the 1980s and early 1990s, chronic fatigue was often referred to dismissively as "Yuppie flu." "Yuppie" is a derogatory term used to denote young, upwardly mobile professionals, middle-class individuals who had forged ahead as bankers and stockbrokers, the privileged and unworthy products of unrestrained profiteering. And at the time it was true that these patients were most commonly the ones seen in fatigue clinics, perhaps (it was sneeringly assumed) because their lack of mental fortitude did not allow them to withstand the pressures of the work from which they profited. Professor Wessely's work showed that in fact the reason middle-class patients were overrepresented in the chronic fatigue service was that they were the ones who had the wherewithal or persistence or ability to get referred to clinics, which at that time were few and far between. But they were not the ones who suffered most; that fate was reserved (as is commonly the case) for people with working-class lives and socioeconomic deprivation, the discovery of which undoubtedly led to an increase in provision of these clinics for the wider population.

Professor Wessely was one of the pioneers of research into chronic fatigue. His research has been extensive, delving into endocrine factors (the study of hormone systems in the body), immunological factors (whether the immune system or antibodies could be influencing fatigue), autonomic function (the nerves that control and regulate bodily functions), as well as the behavioral and psychological aspects of the illness. Patients who saw him in clinic responded to his witty, informal style. One patient used to bake him a cake each time she saw him, so that if you got to clinic early enough on a Tuesday morning, you'd usually be able to take a slice with your cup of tea.

All of this made even more puzzling the extreme reactions from some ME activist groups, who fulminated against him and anything that he said. Over time, the atmosphere has become, if anything, more oppositional. I can think of many researchers in this area who have simply walked away, fed up with the endless jeers, the egregious and willful misrepresentations of them or their work, the weaponization of Freedom of Information requests to undermine and defeat research projects, the vilification of people and research they don't like, and the use of MPs as "useful idiots" to write letters to people in high places in support of their cause, without understanding the issues.

My own experience of this came while I was sitting on a NICE committee. The National Institute for Health and Care Excellence was set up by the British government in 1999 to improve and standardize medical practice throughout England. There were dozens of different types of guidance being produced, from surgery to all branches of medicine, looking at effectiveness and analyzing the cost of treatments. I was invited to sit as an expert on the Chronic Fatigue Guidelines, given my experience in treating patients with this condition. I spent eighteen months sitting on a panel; reading lengthy documents, research papers, and drafts of the guidance; and attending bimonthly meetings, while trying to run my team of three junior doctors, a psychologist, and an assistant psychologist at Guy's Hospital as well as the service at the Maudsley Hospital. The work of writing guidelines can be painful. It was often slow: afternoons could be spent discussing the placement of a comma or rephrasing a sentence that nobody would read. The discussions, often passionate, began to resemble *Monty Python's Life of Brian*, with the bitter arguments between the Judean People's Front and the People's Front of Judea.

At length the lively discussions were knocked into a committee-speak sort of language, denuded of any personality, and published. Still, we had produced what I thought was a useful set of guidelines, a view happily shared by most observers. They were practical and thoughtful and steered a careful path between the strongly held and frequently conflicting views of mainstream medical opinion and those expressed by some patient groups.

As winter set in and the ground hardened under an early frost, I had put the guidelines out of my mind and had started to get on with the hectic rounds of seeing patients, supervising junior doctors, allocating referrals, speaking to GPs, teaching medical students, conducting audits, and the never-ending filling out of electronic forms demanded of the modern doctor. Another email arrived in my inbox, and as usual, unable to find any means of guarding myself against the urge to check on it, instead of finishing what I was doing first, I had a quick peek. Bad idea. It was from a firm of solicitors, always the sort of email to get the pulse quickening. All the problems I've agonized about at length, the difficult clinical or managerial situations, have never in the end caused me too much harm—probably because I've considered and anticipated all the likely eventualities and taken at least some action to guard against problems. My experience is that most bad news simply drops from outer space, unanticipated and shocking.

I didn't really take it in the first time, so I had to reread the email. Activists within the ME community were taking NICE to court for a judicial review of the guidelines. As was made clear to me by NICE's lawyers, it turns out that a person or organization can't object to a set of guidelines written by a public body such as NICE based on the fact that they disagree with the guidelines or simply don't like them. The only avenue open to them, if they wanted to have the guidelines over-turned, was to say that the guideline group itself was constituted with such a bias that no other reasonable body of people could have reached the same conclusions. For this reason, they had to find evidence of bias in the members of the guideline development group, and I was one of the people accused.

The point was to discredit me, so as to discredit the guidelines. The reason I was singled out, along with the psychologist on the committee and a GP, was because I was the only psychiatrist in the guideline group. The involvement of psychiatry is seen as a provocation by people advocating for the diagnosis. I think this is from the notion that because psychological therapies help in the treatment of chronic fatigue syndrome, it implies the illness itself is wholly psychological. It doesn't of course imply anything of the sort. Psychological treatments are helpful in the treatment of a variety of conditions, including diabetes and cardiac problems, although nobody is suggesting that diabetes or heart attacks are mental health conditions.

This debate about the cause of chronic fatigue syndrome, whether it is physical or psychological, is an extension of the Cartesian mind-body split. It is part of our culture that illnesses need to be cast as one or the other, either physical or psychological. But why? Why not both physical *and* psychological? Why can't we accept that illnesses, all illnesses, have varying degrees of physical and psychological components?

I often ask patients whether they have ever had a tension headache. Nearly everyone has. I ask whether they think a tension headache is physical or psychological. On the one hand, we know that tension headaches are caused by stress and tension (hence the name), not by a physical problem such as a brain tumor. So it's psychological, surely? But on the other hand, tension headaches are expressed in a very physical way, with pain, and respond well to physical treatments like paracetamol/acetaminophen. So what is a tension headache? Physical or psychological?

A more fruitless debate is difficult for me to imagine. Anyone who practices medicine, anyone who understands human nature, understands that just about any illness you care to mention has both physical and psychological components. And anyone who has had a tension headache, which is everyone, knows that they really hurt. The pain is not fake, imaginary, or made up; the pain is real and distressing, and it demands action. If the cure is paracetamol, then great, so long as it works quickly. And if the cure is a stress management program, to stop the headaches from recurring, then also great. No need to worry about whether it is physical or psychological. Yet we have become trapped in a way of thinking about illness that causes people to reject treatments that could be helpful, on a matter of principle, and I really can't make sense of that position at all. From my perspective as a clinician, treating patients is about pragmatism, about finding a way. I do not offer treatments based on the elegance of the theory behind the treatment or whether it is consistent with an ideological understanding. I base my treatments on what the evidence shows, what trial data are telling us, and whether it is likely to work.

I support research into a biological understanding of CFS/ME. I hope it will yield new avenues for treatments and cures—a pill, say, that would give immediate relief from the very unpleasant symptoms. But even if it were shown that CFS/ME was partly, predominantly, or even entirely a psychological condition, what would be wrong with that? Why would that make it any less worthy of treatment and research? The implication of this approach is that mental health problems are lesser illnesses and that people with, for example, schizophrenia and depression aren't really suffering. It is as if any suggestion of psychological treatments makes the illness less worthy.

Meanwhile, the legal process ground on. The next stage was that I had to have discussions with lawyers appointed by NICE and then write formal letters defending myself against the charge of bias. The people who brought the case must have overestimated my ability to persuade the other specialists on the panel, including a neurologist, three GPs, an infectious disease specialist, an immunologist, and occupational health specialists, among others. I idly wondered if there was any other branch of medicine where debate about best practice is conducted through law courts, rather than in medical journals.

Eventually, the case went to court, and to say that NICE's victory was emphatic doesn't quite come close to reflecting the displeasure of the judge to whom the case had even been brought at all. Expressed in the cool and precise language of the judiciary, the judgment of Mr. Justice Simon was a masterpiece. He had clearly got all of the nuances and tensions of the debate and concluded with the statement: "First, unfounded as they were, the allegations were damaging to those against whom they were made; and were such as may cause health professionals to hesitate before they involve themselves in this area of medicine. A perception that this is an area of medicine where contrary views are not to be voiced, and where scientific inquiry is to be limited, is damaging to science and harmful to patients." And the tragedy is that I have known a number of fine researchers who have walked away, disillusioned and even broken by the sustained abuse they have received for simply carrying out research for the benefit of the patients they see.

The whole episode left me feeling bruised. I believed that what many people advocating for CFS/ME wanted was for the illness to be taken seriously. The perception was that the only way for it to be taken seriously was to dissociate it from any whiff of psychological contributions, despite the insult this implied to the many people suffering with mental health problems. Yet the split between physical and psychological is nothing more than a reflection of the way medicine is talked about and practiced, so as a profession we are not entirely innocent, and perhaps should not be too surprised that things turned out this way.

Psychiatrists often get accused of talking "psychobabble." I would contend that the opposite happens in this illness. In trying to demonstrate a physical cause, a lot of "biobabble" is talked by doctors who don't really know much about the illness, and who really ought to know better than to be talking about it. "Biobabble" consists of those explanations that sound scientific, that use lots of scientific-sounding words, but that make little scientific sense. Theories are advanced that would embarrass a medical student, let alone a doctor. And as is often the case with all people who don't really know what they are doing, they are certain that they are right. Genuine uncertainty exists in the field, for sure, an uncertainty that I will address with patients. But sometimes patients are more reassured by the certainties of an amateur than by the equivocations of an expert. It brings to mind a quote by the sixteenth-century poet Samuel Daniel: "Whilst timorous Knowledge stands considering / Audacious Ignorance hath done the deede." For now, audacious ignorance abounds in the Wild West of the internet, and worse still, in far too many consulting rooms.

So why did I carry on with this sort of work? Well, the answer was that the thousands of patients whom I have seen over the years have borne with dignity an illness bewildering to them and their families, and which has often had a great impact on their lives. I have never doubted their symptoms or their very real suffering. They come to my clinic to get better, not to promote an ideology of their illness. We have treatments available, treatments far from perfect, but which can provide some measure of relief, and in some cases cure the patient altogether.

The first step in Carole's treatment was to try to make sense of her symptoms, to come to a shared understanding of what was maintaining them, and in light of that, to agree on a way forward. By this time, that was easier said than done. Like a lot of patients I see, she quite understandably wanted every investigation done, some of which I was certain were unnecessary and unhelpful. Over the years that I have been working in this field, I have seen the theories change. For a while, there was a theory that amalgam in fillings was the cause of fatigue, and it was not uncommon for me to see people in clinic with all their fillings replaced with porcelain ones, usually at considerable expense. Enzyme supplements, coenzymes, ever more stringent dietary restrictions, herbs, fish oils, and various actual but inappropriate medications are all part of what a patient may be taking when they first come to see me, despite the lack of evidence to justify their use. At best, many of these treatments are expensive placebos, and at worst, some are actively harmful.

It took some discussion to arrive at a point of mutual understanding with Carole. Whatever caused her symptoms was unknown and in all likelihood will never be known. In the absence of the silver bullet to treat her, we focused on what we could do. It seemed her illness was being maintained by a range of physical and psychological factors, including poor sleep, physical deconditioning, low mood, her relentless focusing on symptoms—and she herself was aware that stress was making things worse, as it does with nearly any health problem. The treatment plan we came up with was in part physical and in part psychological. We came up with an exercise program that gradually and incrementally increased her activity levels, reversing the deconditioning and inconsistent activity that was exacerbating the problem. We developed a sleep program and also explored the role of tension and anxiety in maintaining her problems and her ongoing low mood. Finally, we developed distraction techniques, to reduce the focus on symptoms and health preoccupations, which appeared to maintain her problems. I referred her on to one of the excellent therapists in the unit I work in, who continued the work, seeing her a dozen or so times over the following year.

Little by little, things began to change. The changes were gradual, so improvement came over months. Slowly she started to extend her daily walks and built rest breaks into her routine to avoid the boom-and-bust overactivity followed by exhaustion. Most important, she started to socialize again, to re-engage in life. She took a part-time job in a museum. By the time she was discharged about a year later, she wasn't perfect—she still didn't like to push herself too hard for fear of relapsing—but for the first time in her adult life she was able to manage autonomously and was optimistic about the future. The last time I saw her, she didn't see me, because she was out with friends at a café in Camberwell as I happened to be walking past. She was holding court at the center of the table, and the sounds of her laughter made me realize that I had never heard it before.

SUICIDE

Over my career I have assessed many thousands of patients and would estimate that about a quarter to a half have considered suicide. Most of those people are horrified by the thought that they would actually act on any suicidal impulses, and some tell me that they even take an extra step backward on a train platform when a train goes past, just to be sure that they couldn't act on any urge to jump. Other patients I see have a still more ambivalent attitude toward life and death. I have had patients tell me they deliberately don't look when crossing the road, letting fate decide if they get knocked down or not. I had one patient who would turn the lights off in her car while driving at night on the pitch-black countryside roads near her home, not exactly trying to crash, but not exactly trying not to. I find this ambivalence toward life quite common. Sometimes people within the same consultation will tell me about both their plan to visit a relative in another part of the country next and their imminent plan of suicide. Obviously both things can't be true. This can mean that a clinical consultation is difficult to make sense of, because the messages are mixed and frequently the patients themselves are not sure what they want.

Ambivalence is commonly at the heart of suicidal impulses and is often reflected in such contradictory behaviors. A person can both want to die and want to live, which is why, blown like a reed in the wind, chance happenings can either pull them back from the brink of suicide or firm their resolve. My experience is that most people really want to live, not to die, but they want to live a different life, one free from the emotional pain of the one that they are living. The suicide attempt is made in the hope that as a result, something will change, and with a single bound they will be freed of their emotional burdens. This is sometimes dismissed as a "cry for help," which trivializes the profound mental anguish that leads people to this point, although the term does capture something of the inner mental process. I have also, it must be said, had patients under my care who have attempted suicide and have been stopped from doing so at the last minute, or have been found at home by an unexpected visitor, or have been resuscitated in the hospital. In these situations, the drive for suicide was implacable and determined, and only luck stood in their way. Thankfully I have never had a patient manage to kill himself or herself, although it has happened to patients in the care of my psychiatry team, for which I am ultimately responsible.

Many factors make suicide more likely. Being alone, lacking a family or friends or a network of support, increases the likelihood of suicide. Older age increases risk, so that while I take suicidal thoughts seriously regardless of the age of the person telling me about them, I am especially wary when an older adult reveals suicidal thoughts. Being unemployed or having a chronic illness (either mental or physical) compounds the risk of suicide. I suspect that these things amplify a sense of detachment from society, which is never healthy. Loneliness is a rising epidemic in our culture. In the United States, it is estimated that up to 47 percent of adults are lonely, a figure that is considered to present the same risk as smoking fifteen cigarettes a day. One study reported that over 9 million adults in the UK are often or always lonely, almost a fifth of the population. A poignant, even haunting statistic is that the charity Age UK estimates that television or pets are the main form of company for almost half (49 percent) of adults over sixty-five. I worry about the effects of loneliness on the mental health of the population, because we are fundamentally social beings. Having a connection to a community protects against the development of both physical and mental health problems. Belonging to a church or a cricket club or even just being a regular at the local pub or part of the darts team—all of these increase our connectedness to a community and are healthy for us.

We tend to assume that so far as health is under our control, it relates to diet and alcohol and exercise, and we give little thought to the value of our social connections. Yet doing things for others and being part of something bigger than yourself are not just good ways to improve self-esteem and mental health; they improve our physical health, too. I have often wondered how good mental health improves our resistance to illness. It is at least plausible that it works via the immune system, a notion that has generated some research interest and chimes with our everyday experience. We have all had that feeling of being stressed, for example, and stress lowers our resistance to catching infections. At the more extreme end, one often-cited paper speculated that chronic stress, via its effects on the immune system, might promote the initiation and progression of some types of cancer.

Related to social cohesion, there is good evidence that racism in society affects not only mental health but physical health as well. An editorial in the *British Medical Journal* reported that victims of racism were more likely to have a limiting long-term illness, high blood pressure, and respiratory disease. There is evidence from a study in the United States that racism causes increased mortality rates not just in the black community but perhaps surprisingly in the white population, too. Even if you are not the victim, there is something toxic about racism. Not only does it impoverish and poison our society, but it is biologically toxic to the human body. There are no clear explanations as to why social cohesion is protective or racism promotes illness. Our biologically centered approach to an understanding of the human body means that physical illness developing as a result of social adversity or a lack of social cohesion does not intuitively make sense. But after twenty years of seeing these sorts of correlations, I have stopped being surprised by them.

Society also plays other roles in influencing suicide risk. Prior to 1961, suicide attempts in the UK were actually a criminal offense. While this may seem absurd, and people may reasonably ask what kind of deterrent a criminal sanction is to someone who is dead, it did in my view send a powerful message that suicide is a societal taboo. There is good evidence from more than one study that copycat suicides spike after a suicide is shown on television, particularly when the character is portrayed as having impossible choices to make and seeing no alternative. Very quickly people come to empathize with the character and see suicide as an alternative solution to their own desperate life situations. I think the taboo around suicide here can be protective.

The counterargument is that criminalizing suicide is heartless. Worse, though, it may be actively promoting suicide because it stops people from talking about the thoughts that drive them to such a desperate act. One of the biggest complaints from the suicidal people I have treated is that they feel isolated, afraid to discuss their thoughts with anyone for fear of what people might think or say. These kinds of taboos can be fatal. If the end result of removing the stigma around the discussion of suicide is to reduce the suicide rate, then we need to be able to talk about these things without emotion or drama or the threat of criminal prosecution.

Interestingly, one of the most effective ways to reduce suicide is to remove the means of suicide. Some years back, a common method of suicide in the UK was by inhalation of toxic gases used in home ovens. People would put their head in the oven and inhale the gases. But after the switch from coal gas to the less toxic North Sea gas, this method stopped being lethal. What was interesting was that there was a transient dip in the number of suicides, as people attempted suicide unsuccessfully. Yet there was no increase of suicide afterward. You might think that if a person attempts suicide and the attempt is unsuccessful, they'll just try again, but it is not as simple as that. It seems that if you can remove the means of carrying out a potentially lethal act, then the person might go on to have many more years of life ahead of them. This is one reason motorways and "suicide bridges" have protective fencing around them, to avoid impulsive attempts to jump from bridges and buy some time for the suicidal impulse to subside. For the same reason, wards in hospitals have ligature points (anything that can be used to attach a cord or rope, or other means of hanging or strangulation) removed; and there is evidence that blister packs of tablets reduce suicide rate compared with bottles. With a bottle of tablets, you can tip all the tablets out into your hand at once, whereas with blister packs it takes time to pop each tablet individually into your hand, so fewer tablets can be grabbed and taken impulsively. By the time enough tablets have been taken out to make the overdose dangerous, just enough time may have elapsed for the individual to start having second thoughts. Similarly, gun laws that restrict the availability of firearms will reduce the suicide rate. The ease of use, lethality, and availability of guns in some countries lead to a significant risk of impulsive suicide. In the United States, studies have shown a strong link between overall state firearm ownership and firearm suicide. And so, at least in part, my role as a psychiatrist when I see suicidal patients is to get them beyond the crisis, in the hope that the blue skies will once again appear, and a life will be saved.

People's attitudes toward their own lives can be difficult to understand and built on shifting sands. I remember treating Anton, who was born into a working-class family and was prodigiously bright. He had an academic career that took him to the University of Cambridge to read economics—he was the first person from his school ever to go there—and his school was justifiably proud of him. He got a first-class degree and then moved to a banking job in the City of London and started to build a career. But he never really felt like the others. He said that he didn't fit into their social circle, but instead felt like the working-class boy who didn't belong. After one bad week, in which he had lost money for the bank in a series of trades, he started to doubt himself. It was clearly hard for him to talk about this. He cried at this point in his retelling and had to stop, then wept more or less continually as the interview wore on, apologizing all the time.

One of the few constants in my job is the fact that people feel the need to apologize when they cry. I told Anton that having emotions is part of being human. Sometimes the emotions are sadness and tears, sometimes happiness and laughter, and there's no need to apologize for tears any more than for laughing at a joke. But Anton sat there—cheeks wet, nose running—looking helpless.

He continued his story. He said that after his bad week he became more obsessional, found it increasingly hard to make decisions, and isolated himself from his coworkers. He worked longer hours, but this did not help his decision-making, which, if anything, became worse. He began to feel useless at work, and his mood started to deteriorate further. He lost his appetite, stopped sleeping properly, and felt exhausted and demotivated. It was after another sleepless night that he had made a basic but very costly error, putting the decimal point in the wrong place in a trade. His boss at that point said that he needed to take a break. Anton read into this that he was going to be fired, and he felt a terrible shame, fearful that he had let everyone down throughout his life, all those who had supported him at school and at home.

When I saw him in my outpatient department, he was unhappy, anxious, and uncertain and had developed many features of depression. Underpinning this was a self-esteem that had never been very high in the first place, and which was now in the basement. He believed that he was a failure, a social misfit, and that the only reason he had been allowed to rise so high was so that people could take pleasure in his subsequent fall. He admitted that he had been having regular and intrusive thoughts of death and dying and had started to wonder whether suicide would be an option. He had researched suicide methods on the internet and maintained that the people who had held him back from considering suicide before, his family and friends, no longer provided the same restraint. He thought killing himself might be kinder for them than having someone around who was a burden and a source of shame.

I have been down this road with patients many times before and know that it can be very hard to roll back the situation all at once. Most cases involve three steps, the first of which is to avoid a suicide while the treatment in steps two and three are under way. This first step is always a delicate one, as it is not a single action. By listening carefully and being able to summarize their problem back to them, you demonstrate to the patient that you understand their predicament. It is important not to offer judgments, by word or gesture, no matter what your personal views of suicide are. At the same time, you need to be able to handle the situation. You can't start getting teary, flustered, or angry, nor can you exhibit any other emotion that may pass through your mind, no matter how tragic or distressing the situation or how senseless the patient's actions appear to you. The patient has told you something that has been told to nobody else, and it has taken great courage for them to do so. They do not need to see their psychiatrist struggling to cope (that is precisely, of course, why they have not told their family).

Don't shoot from the hip. Some problems don't have quick and easy solutions. A mistake that I see junior doctors regularly make is to offer reassurance far too early, in an attempt to show compassion and support. Unfortunately, however well intentioned, to patients this is rarely reassuring. To be told that "everything is going to be fine" is not convincing to anyone, unless you can back it up with a well-argued and convincing reason why. You need to be able to instill in the patient some sense of hope for the future, and this has to be based on the consultation that you have had, so that it is grounded in reality. And finally, the great intangible is to transmit to the patient that you care about what happens. The patient needs to be forming this impression throughout the interview and arrive at this conclusion themselves. This is a skill that in my experience can't be taught, because patients can always tell, through all the verbal and nonverbal communications, exactly who is interested in them and who is not. And for all of that, I still make backup plans and give the patient numbers to call in a crisis.

The second step is treating the depression. Some honesty with patients is required here. Choice of antidepressants is based on trial data, of course, but a given antidepressant does not work in every patient, for reasons nobody fully understands. Matters are complicated by the unpredictable way in which patients will tolerate some antidepressants but not others. Finding the right treatment can take a bit of patience, and it can take two or three attempts before the right medication or combination of medications is found. In Anton's case, I tried one antidepressant that he had to stop because of side effects, a second that was not particularly effective, and a third, which he said after a few weeks was starting to take effect ("I'm like a drowning man coming up for air"). Once he was able to think more clearly, not weighted down by his depression, it was time to try to unravel a lifetime of unwarranted low self-esteem (step three). This process is something like a barrister asking questions of a witness in court. What you are trying to do is to move the patient into a position where they see their low self-esteem as illogical, an unwarranted emotion not supported by the facts. ("So despite your first-class degree in economics from the University of Cambridge, you believe that everyone is cleverer than you?") It involves challenging notions such as the idea that making a mistake makes you a failure, something that preoccupied Anton. (I quoted a half-remembered line from *The Simpson's*: "But doesn't everyone make mistakes? Isn't that why they put an eraser on the top of pencils?") Specific events are analyzed and the individual's reactions to them reviewed, to see if their emotions are supported by the facts of the situation.

We all have biases in our thinking. With medical students I often try the following: Imagine if I told you that you were a good medical student, but your knowledge of pharmacology needed work. Some of you would feel pretty pleased with yourselves. ("He said I was a good medical student. I'm cruising here.") Others would start to read failure into it. ("He was trying to butter me up with the 'good medical student' thing. But that was only to soften the blow of what he really wanted to say, which is that I'm not good enough. I knew I couldn't do pharmacology. It'll come up in the exam and I'll fail it. I should have listened to everyone who told me I couldn't cope at medical school.") I point out that one single objective statement has been interpreted in vastly divergent ways depending on one's personality and style, in one case leading to angst and depression, in the other to tranquility and self-satisfaction. It's not the objective reality that leads to depression and self-doubt; it's the subjective interpretation of reality that does it.

These biases in our thinking are well known. People with low self-esteem can have a reflex tendency to dismiss positive comments about themselves ("They were just being nice") and become preoccupied by negative comments ("You see? That's probably what everyone thinks about me"). The problem is that these thinking biases, automatic and unchallenged, become the basis on which emotions are built. If patients can be taught to think more rationally and logically about their circumstances, they can start to align their emotions with the logic of a situation rather than just jump to unwarranted conclusions based on biased thinking.

It's an impossible task to do this work when someone is severely depressed, because their thoughts are so skewed by their low mood that they are unable to really engage in a logical discussion. Gradually, though, Anton was able to start working through the thinking biases that had had such a negative effect on his mood. All of this took time, many weeks, but the plan held together, and he gradually emerged from the situation, shocked by how his own thinking processes had let him down and led him to the brink of suicide. He reflected, when we met at a later appointment, that the worst sort of mental anguish is caused by not knowing whether you can rely on your own thoughts, and to what extent your thoughts might be deceiving you. I think that was particularly galling for him, because his mind was the very basis of his success and advancement so far in life, only to become suddenly unreliable, the thing that had undermined him and brought him to the very depths of despair. That morning alone in my clinic, Anton was the third person I had seen who had been contemplating suicide. Each person has experienced a whole lifetime of events and decisions that have led them to that point. It is the commonest cause of death for men under fifty, and each day at work I try to hold back the tide of sadness and despair that washes in.

Sometimes the tidal wave threatens to engulf me. There are times when a patient's story is so moving that it can be hard to let it go. I feel drained and exhausted. I try to resist feeling too much, for fear that it may be difficult to contain my emotions. I think of the patient I saw with such severe depression that he developed auditory hallucinations, voices telling him he was worthless, whispering in his ear that the least he could do was kill himself. When he came to see me, his head was bandaged after he had tried to cut his ear off. He didn't think he could face any more life. Who would have blamed him? I shudder, force the image from my head, but then I see the woman from Sierra Leone who had been traumatized by the civil war, who had seen her family murdered in front of her. I see her quiet dignity, her tears glistening as she recounts how she had been raped, and I want her to stop. But she must go on, and I must listen, wondering as well how she can carry on with life.

They are now my responsibility. Their death, if they attempt suicide, will be my failure, yet not one over which I have control. How can I control the patient's flashbacks, their desperation, their drinking at night to numb the pain—all those things that push them closer to the brink? I cannot. I must instead control my own anxieties, my own emotions. I must make a plan, take a breath, call the next patient in.

WEIGHT

It was obvious only in retrospect that I was headed for a career in psychiatry, yet the clues were there throughout my childhood. I remember my older sister subscribing to teen magazines, first *Jackie* and then *My Guy*. Occasionally the newsagent would deliver *Blue Jeans* magazine instead, another of the huge stable of teen magazines prevalent in that era, without any explanation. He presumably felt them to be, with some justification, interchangeable. Not wanting to be caught reading any such magazine, wary of the teasing and hilarity it would provoke, I would intercept the post before it had been picked up off the doormat and read the magazines from cover to cover. I would start with the photo love stories; assiduously study the horoscope in the hope that it portended a romance for the twelve-year-old me; then flick through the full-page pictures of Leif Garrett, the elaborately coiffed teen idol, or those of other teen heartthrobs. Finally it was on to my favorite page, the problem page, with the advice columnists Cathy and Claire. I would read each problem, covering up Cathy and Claire's advice while I considered and then wrote down my own solution, which I would then compare with theirs. I nodded sympathetically at the betrayals of fickle boyfriends and best friends, yet was prepared to dish out some hard truths. To others I would gently explain that he doesn't love you, but rather is using you to get to your best friend, as would be obvious if you reread your question. Overbearing parents, acne, strange smells, the first kiss (of which I had at that stage only theoretical knowledge), bullying, exclusion, mean teachers, lecherous teachers, overfamiliar parental friends, inadequate pocket money—all of these problems would merit a considered response, kept in a little notebook, as I built a database of life's teen difficulties.

Among the letters and bills and the teen magazines were also weight-loss magazines, to which my mother subscribed. I would marvel at how so many found space on the newsagent's shelf. It was difficult to see what these magazines could find to say in every issue, when weight loss seemed to me such a straightforward problem. Yes, I could understand the human-interest stories ("Doctors said I had only three months to live!"), which invariably included a photograph of a smiling individual wearing her old jeans, her arms outstretched, gripping the fabric of the denim now feet away from her body, to demonstrate her dramatic weight loss. But it seemed to me then that weight loss was a simple mathematical equation—calories in minus calories expended. The complexities of weight gain, and all the associated psychological baggage and misery, were another world. It seemed, to me at least, that no one else was talking about the psychological aspects of weight gain. The magazines included an endless parade of different diets and recipes, each fad diet cloaked in a pseudoscientific garb, with plenty of mentions of words like "amino acids," "nutrient cycles," and "metabolism," the furious and desperate use of which hid the poverty of the science behind them. The diets all contained a fundamental paradox (the holy grail of diets): you could eat as much you wanted, never be hungry, yet still lose weight. To my younger self, these diet magazines were confusing, point-less, and faintly ridiculous.

The obesity crisis had yet to fully develop in the UK when I was at medical school, although in the United States it was just starting to take hold. When I lecture about obesity, I usually start by referencing the U.S. Centers for Disease Control and Prevention (CDC) data, showing the alarming increase in rates of obesity in the United States over the period of time from 1985 to 2010. Obesity levels are calculated for each of the fifty states. In 1990, no state in the U.S. had obesity levels of over 15 percent. Two decades later, in 2010, no state had obesity levels under 20 percent. In thirty-six states, the rates of obesity were over 25 percent. The rise in obesity levels is indicated by colors on the map of each state, with increasing rates of obesity colored a darker shade of red. This provides a striking visual image of the year-by-year worsening of the crisis.

At medical school, we were given little information about obesity as a looming public health threat. When obesity was mentioned, it was in the context of a dry and unemotional analysis of the increased risks of certain diseases that obesity conferred. We were told next to nothing about the psychological aspects of eating and obesity. In my years as a medical student, I can remember hearing discussed only a single study on this topic, a study that I have since hunted for and never been able to find. Because it was unusual, it stuck in my mind. In the study, subjects were told that their heartbeat was being picked up by sensors in the room and would be played back to them by means of speakers in the corners of the room. Yet there were no sensors picking up the subject's heart rate. Instead, recordings of heart rhythms were played through the speakers—sometimes normal; sometimes dangerous-sounding fast and irregular heart rhythms, to alarm the subject. Placed around the room in which the subjects were listening to what they believed was their heartbeat were bowls of cashew nuts. What the experimenters found was that overweight individuals, when alarmed by the fast and irregular heartbeat, which they thought was signifying something dangerous happening to their bodies, would start eating the cashews from the bowl as a way to calm their anxieties. Normal weight subjects did not do that. This was the first insight I had into the emotional aspects of eating. My own experience, when I had exams or other anxieties at medical school, was that the last thing I wanted to do was to eat. Before I took a set of exams, eating became a dutiful chore, and I might as well have been eating cotton wool for all the pleasure it gave me.

A few years after I started working at Guy's Hospital, a weight-loss service, known medically as a bariatric service, was set up. It was a new approach, reflecting the obesity epidemic starting to take hold in the UK. I was asked to assess the suitability for surgery of those people who had been unable to lose weight on the various diets they had been given. In my training in psychiatry I hadn't come across this kind of situation before, so I wrote to different centers in the United States asking for their advice, and received helpful protocols that they used for their assessments, which I then adapted for the UK.

A trickle of referrals quickly became a stream, although I remember the first patient, Terry, well. He walked into my consulting room, and as he sat down, I noticed that the only chair in the room for him to sit on was narrow, with wooden armrests on each side. He didn't mention it and neither did I, but I was aware of his spilling out of the sides of the chair and thought about his discomfort as we discussed the events that had brought him to see me. Terry came from a seaside town in the north of England. He told me about his childhood, brought up in an impoverished but loving family. He was happy in his childhood, played football on the streets near his house after school, and had a small circle of friends. Life ticked along normally until one day, out of the blue, his older brother was accused of rape. Nobody believed that he could have done such a thing, yet inevitably there was gossip and speculation. The wheels of justice turned slowly, and although the charges were eventually dropped before the case reached trial, his family buckled under the pressure. His father started drinking and became increasingly erratic and bad tempered at home, and when that behavior extended to his work, he lost his job as a cashier in one of the pier amusement arcades. Everyone at Terry's school seemed to know what had happened, both to his accused brother and his drunken father. He was teased and bullied. One boy at school said to him that his family consisted of "a saddo and a sicko." He became withdrawn and increasingly isolated. It wasn't long before he discovered that eating gave him some fleeting pleasure and satisfaction, offering a brief respite from his daily unhappiness. He ate bags of crisps and chocolate bars, ice cream and doughnuts, sweets, marshmallows, jelly beans, and anything else that came to hand. As he got heavier and heavier, the bullying got worse (at school he was now known as Ten-Ton Terry), his isolation increased, and the cycle of weight gain continued.

What struck me as he spoke was not what he was saying but how eager he was to talk. I had assumed patients in this clinic would find seeing a psychiatrist off-putting, a hurdle to overcome in their path to get weight-loss surgery. Yet the experience I had with this patient was exactly the opposite. A lifetime of being marginalized had made him lonely. He had few opportunities to speak to someone interested in what he had to say, and his self-esteem was almost nonexistent. He lived alone, had few friends, had never had a girlfriend, and had never had a sexual relationship, something he seemed relieved to discuss with me, to try to normalize what for him was a millstone around his neck.

Terry had just turned thirty-one when I saw him, and his life seemed to be going nowhere. He had not had a long-term job in his life, but would take on occasional work where he could get it. Whenever he did have work, his attendance record was patchy, and he would usually end up being fired. Terry, however, attributed the loss of his job to a lack of competence rather than to his spotty attendance, which served only to worsen his self-esteem. In keeping with this, he started but never saw through diets, giving up after days or weeks. His life was lived largely on his own. He had some contact with his family, but he was now in London and they were on the coast. He told me that food was the only thing in life he really enjoyed, and he used it to deal with any emotion. Thinking of the "cashew nut" study from medical school, I asked him if it helped with anxiety. He told me it did, and he told me that he found it hard to differentiate now between feelings of anxiety and the feeling of hunger. He only knew that eating calmed his anxieties. Yet his anxiety was not the only emotion that led him to eat. He said that he would eat in response to anger, frustration, sadness, boredom, happiness, or any other emotion that he experienced.

Bariatric surgery was obviously not going to resolve the problems that had led him to this stage in his life. While an operation might immediately help with weight loss, he was unlikely to sustain the weight loss if the issues that caused this eating pattern were not addressed. As we both stood up at the end of the consultation, he towered above me. He was wearing dirty, loose-fitting, thin gray jogging pants that had lost their shape. There were food stains on the hoodie that he wore, and as soon as he left the consultation, he put the hood up, although it wasn't particularly cold. He seemed to shrink, his shoulders rounded and hunched, as if he were trying to hide from the world around him. I had overrun the appointment by at least twenty minutes, something I rarely do, but he just wanted to keep talking. I sensed he was not normally a talkative person. The waiting room when I got there was restless, and since I dislike running late, I just got on with my clinic, only thinking about Terry when I came to dictate his letter later that afternoon, once clinic had ended.

A few weeks later I saw Lena in one of my outpatient clinics. Lena weighed over 300 pounds, and at five and a half feet tall, had a body mass index of 48. A healthy body mass index is in the range of 18 to 25, and obesity is defined as anything over 30. My first thought as I saw Lena was that she looked quite depressed. Head bowed, making little eye contact, she moved effortfully into my clinic room. As we moved down the corridor, she all but ignored my usual small talk. By then, after my experience with Terry, I had made sure the department ordered some more comfortable chairs, and this had happened surprisingly quickly. So added to my array of mismatched clinic room furniture was a large chair in a dun color that had a faintly institutional air about it. I remembered it was still in the corner of the clinic room, not positioned across from my desk, so I scuttled ahead of Lena as we made our way down the corridor, managing to rearrange the chairs before she arrived at the door. She sat down heavily, then half lifted her head to take in her surroundings. Because of her size, I assumed she was older than she was—only thirty-eight, as it turned out.

Lena had been born in Poland and had lived there until her mid-twenties. She came from a small town in the north of the country. She was the oldest of seven children. Her religious parents were born and had grown up in the same town, with no ambition to leave. Her mother worked as a nurse and her father as an electrician. They contributed their spare time to the local church community and were content with their lives. She remembered it as a quiet town. She said that her family never went on vacation, as there was not enough money. Occasionally there would be day trips to the seaside, but as the oldest sibling, she didn't have anyone to talk to—her brothers were too young and immature, her parents too old—so she sulked for most of those outings, not wanting to be with her family, but not wanting to be at home either. When I asked her what she remembered most clearly about her childhood, she recalled being bored. She said that at school she was an average student: she enjoyed art but was not particularly good at sport or in academic subjects. She was popular, though, and was generally considered to be very pretty. She remembered the boys all wanting to dance with her and ask her out, and she enjoyed the feeling this gave her. It offered her some excitement and an escape away from what she considered her restricted and humdrum small-town life.

She left school as soon as she could. She had no interest in higher education. Her parents were disappointed, but Lena wanted to earn her own money and to live a more eventful and exciting life. The first job she got was as a waitress in a diner. She loved it there. She enjoyed chatting with the customers, flirting a little, and having some disposable income for her evenings out. She remembered one evening, a Friday night. She was working the late shift, and she had been serving a table of six men in their early twenties, perhaps slightly older. They had been a bit forward with her, but she felt she knew how to take care of herself. One of the men arranged to meet her when her shift ended, and since she fancied him, she was not against the idea of a little adventure.

I tried to imagine what the diner looked like—perhaps a Polish version of something distinctively American. I imagined it too brightly lit, Formica tables with plastic stools nailed into the floor; a little sad, somewhat desperate. I tried to visualize what she might have looked like as a younger woman. She had quite striking eyes, but whereas they once may have been playful, they now had a sadness in them. Her lip trembled and she reached for the box of tissues on the corner of the desk. She cried, blew her nose, and I waited for her to finish, thinking of her walking out of an overbright Polish diner, knowing what she was going to say next.

She met up with him at the end of her shift, in a car park. I don't know why I imagined pine trees around the car park, and I knew it couldn't be correct, but the image came into my mind unbidden, of her walking along dried pine needles, the scent of a summer's evening giving way to the cool of night as she walked with him to his van. He attacked her, raped her, and her life then had a before and an after, an event that defined her life and divided it into two.

She couldn't tell anyone what had happened, least of all her parents. She felt deeply ashamed, and her religious upbringing found expression only in her guilt. She blamed herself, somehow saw herself as the seducer, even though she had been attacked. She decided that she no longer wanted to have romance and relationships in her life, having experienced the brutal consequences. She did not want men to look at her anymore. She withdrew from life, spending more time at home and no longer looking at herself in the mirror. Her weight steadily climbed, which she saw as good, a deterrent against unwanted attention. And so life continued, passing her by as she took a series of temporary jobs.

She came to the UK, and as her English improved, she got a job in a call center. Having a sedentary job did little to help her lose weight. In fact, she grew heavier, to the extent that she developed joint pains and sleep apnea, making her fatigued during the day. When she started showing signs of prediabetes, she was referred into a weight management program. She had by then failed on several diets, and a surgical option was proposed as the only way she was likely to lose enough weight for her health to improve.

She saw herself as having failed in life. She felt she had not been a good daughter or a good Catholic. She was convinced she would never be a wife or mother, and saw life now as only something to be endured, in pain and in poor health. A diagnosis of depression did not seem to capture the complex emotions and self-loathing that had resulted in her coming to see me.

I was briefly lost in a reverie as I wrote up my notes. As a junior doctor in internal medicine, when I got up in the morning for a sixty-hour shift on call, I would wonder if at that very moment a middle-aged man was experiencing the first tightening in his chest, and our paths would cross later that day as he arrived in casualty. I was taken by the idea of an inescapable destiny, that for a brief moment in time, his life and mine would become briefly entangled before once again returning to our own separate destinies. I wondered about the same thing with Lena right then. I thought back to what I was doing at each of the times she described, until the lines representing our lives crossed at this very moment. I wondered if I would be up to it, whether I was going to make her any better.

"Will you have to section me?"

I was startled out of my reverie. I put my pen down and looked up at her. A section, an involuntary committal to a psychiatric facility, was such an outlandish possibility that it hadn't crossed my mind that she could be worried about that. Invoking a section of the Mental Health Act to compel treatment is something reserved for the most dire and worrisome cases, not for someone struggling to lose weight. I must have misheard.

"I'm sorry. Will I what?"

"Will you have to section me?" she whispered, and burst into tears again.

I felt a real sympathy for her. I realized that for her to have told me the things she did, believing that at the end of it she might have been compelled to have an admission to a psychiatric ward, was an act of bravery. I tried to reassure her. "Even if we had a bed to put you in, which I don't think we've had in weeks, there's absolutely no chance I'd be putting you in it." Despite myself I couldn't help laughing at the thought, and that seemed to unlock something in her. She began to laugh and cry at the same time. It was not until a few minutes later, after lots of noisy nose blowing, that we could get on with the business at hand.

It was clear, both in Lena's case and in Terry's, that an operation was not going to solve the problem, or at least not on its own. Weight-loss surgery before someone is psychologically prepared for it is a fool's errand, likely to end in failure and sometimes disaster. This can mean simply that the surgery doesn't achieve its desired effect and the patient doesn't lose weight or loses some and quickly puts it back on. Sometimes the consequences are more serious, like stomach pain and bloating, regret and depression. Some patients still manage to eat after they feel full, especially high-calorie foods that melt, like ice cream or chocolate. It's especially easy to drink your calories. One study found an increased suicide rate in the ten years after bariatric surgery.

So an understanding of the psychological issues is key, and sometimes the intervention can be straightforward. I remember one man who was unable to lose weight, and when I asked about what he was eating and why he was putting weight on, he said he was eating too much cake and too many biscuits and crisps.

"But I thought you lived alone," I said. "So who is buying all this stuff?"

"Well, my nephew sometimes comes over and he likes a treat."

"But why does he have to eat it at your house?"

"I've got friends who come round. What would I serve them? What would they think?"

"But if they're friends of yours, wouldn't they want to support your diet? I'm sure they'd want that more than they'd want to have a slice of cake when they came to your house."

The message got through, because when I next saw him, he said he was starting to lose weight and wasn't sure he wanted the surgery anymore. He had come to the realization that once food was in his shopping basket, it was a question of when, and not whether, he would eat it. It came to him like a flash of insight, although in fact I had been trying to explain that very thing to him at the previous appointment.

But with Terry and with Lena, it was a different story. For them, food and obesity were just symptoms of a deeper unhappiness in their lives, and weight-loss surgery on its own was never going to remedy that. I had several more appointments with Terry, helping him identify and understand his emotions so that he could have a more considered response to his feelings than just turning to food. He learned to differentiate between actual hunger and emotional hunger. We actively looked for better ways to deal with his emotions, because you can't just remove eating as a means of coping without replacing it with something else. Eating is a behavior, the outward manifestation of inner distress, that eventually becomes self-perpetuating. Someone can't stop a long-standing habit or behavior through effort of will. These are behaviors that have been built up over years, often in response to feelings of inadequacy, unhappiness, or other such emotions, and sustained by routine, habit, helplessness, and despair. A way has to be found to normalize the relationship with food, at the same time ensuring the old eating patterns are not replaced by a different and equally unhelpful way of coping with emotion, such as smoking or using drugs.

Helping him identify his feeling was stage one; rebuilding his life was stage two. After the first stage he was ready for the surgery, which he had with some success. Yet it was hard to unravel a lifetime of insecurity and feelings of worthlessness. It was also difficult to try to build a life for someone with no stable job, no friends, and few interests. He started to lose weight and feel better about himself, yet was isolated and lonely, and I worried he was at risk of slipping back into the old patterns of behavior that had led him to see me in the first place. He was timid in his social life, reluctant to apply for jobs, and scared of getting into relationships. He kept referring to his low self-esteem, by which he really meant an anxiety about being rejected, this being the story of his whole life, and which put him off doing anything at all. It was a slow process, helping him set realistic goals and head toward the targets he had set for his work and social life.

Despite my best-laid plans, his most significant improvement came about in a way that had almost nothing to do with me. He mentioned to me at one outpatient appointment that he was thinking of buying a dog, which I absent-mindedly said sounded to me like a perfectly good idea. Yet even I could not have foreseen how much this decision would change him. He felt a responsibility for his (surprisingly small) dog. He would enthusiastically show me pictures of it on his phone, doing all the sorts of unremarkable things that dogs do. He walked it each day and eventually fell into conversation with other dog owners. When I discharged him, he was in a fledgling relationship, he had maintained his weight loss, and for the first time he could recall, he was looking forward with optimism to the future.

Lena, too, needed preparation if she was going to have surgery, but her case was altogether more challenging. She was a likable woman, yet she had come to use food as a means of keeping the world at arm's length. It took a little time for her to see it that way, however apparent it might have been to an outside observer. Her biggest issue was that she had never really developed any relationships. I was worried about what would happen to her postoperatively, when she no longer had her weight to protect her. How would she begin to form normal and more intimate bonds? How would she understand and cope with the feelings of guilt, shame, and failure lingering from her childhood and early adulthood? For her, surgery was just the beginning of the story, not the happy ending in itself.

I referred her for cognitive analytical therapy, a form of treatment halfway between cognitive behavioral therapy and psychoanalysis. The treatment involved an exploration of her relationships and family dynamics, looking for the explanations as to why she felt the emotions that she felt, but also tied in with more practical solutions to her behavior in the future. When I last saw her, some months after the operation, she was certainly slimmer, but in regard to her life and relationships, she was a work in progress. What troubled her was not simply the assault, but the associated beliefs that she was a bad person and had encouraged and possibly deserved what had happened to her. These ideas are difficult to hear, particularly when they fly in the face of all reason. Nobody ever deserves to be assaulted, and the blame must lie with the perpetrator. Yet we are not rational observers of our lives: we all have contradictory and often irrational beliefs about ourselves and the world around us, many of which defy logic, but which go unchallenged throughout our lives. Sometimes these beliefs help us—for example, when we persist and succeed despite our shortcomings—and sometimes they come to constrain and define us, as they did with Lena.

During a career spent in psychiatry, I have found that there is no better teacher in life than time in understanding human nature, and thus in understanding our patients. The boxer Mike Tyson famously said: "Everyone has a plan until they get punched in the mouth." All of us can moralize about weight, give unsolicited advice, and criticize others. It's only when life delivers you a fierce punch, one that leaves you rocking on your feet, that you realize that you, too, are vulnerable and insecure. When people think of obesity, they commonly think of individuals lacking in self-control, weak people lacking in moral fiber. They imagine that by an effort of will, simply by exerting better self-control, those individuals will be able to lose weight. Many obese patients tell me that they are aware that others think this, and in fact they themselves internalize these thoughts. They begin to see themselves in the same way as others see them, as lazy and weak-willed, and this makes them feel even worse. Yet the drivers for eating and obesity are complex. Undoubtedly there is a genetic component to obesity—there nearly always is with any complex trait. But just as someone's height can be altered by factors like malnutrition or illness, so obesity is far more than a function of just the genetic factors. Pricing and availability of food both matter. Eating healthily can be much more expensive than eating filling, high-calorie food such as burgers and doughnuts. Psychological factors make a substantive difference as well, both in causing the obesity in the first place and then in contributing to the sense of defeatism and despair that accompanies it. Without an understanding of the psychological, how can we hope to understand the physical problems with which they present? And more important, how can we hope to treat them? I think back to my childhood, the weight-loss magazines stacked on the living room shelf, and I think back to my great-aunt Pearl and the weight problems that beset and eventually defined her. I feel that life has made me sadder, wiser, and far slower to pass judgment. Medicine without wisdom is worth nothing at all.

BELIEF

My grandmother would stay at our house when my parents were away when I was a child—my grandfather had long since died. My grandmother's family, so far as she knew, came from Romania and Russia, arriving in the United Kingdom some time around 1900, to the northern town of Sheffield. In one branch of the family tree there was a long line of rabbis, and she would tell me about the strict rules she had to adhere to when she visited her own grandparents on the Sabbath as a girl—no adjusting lights, no writing, no cooking. ("If there was any bubbling of the stew in the oven on Sabbath, my grandmother wouldn't eat it. She would drink lemonade and eat challah all day.") My grandmother was brought up in England, although she also spoke Yiddish, a rich and expressive language that would pepper her conversation. In an attempt to capture a feeling in a way that she couldn't in English, she would frequently lapse into the language, so I grew up with a smattering of Yiddish words and expressions, some of which I didn't realize weren't English until I was at university.

My grandmother would cook heavy, starchy broths thickened with cornstarch, puddings, gravy, and potato latkes. She would hover over my siblings and me as we ate, taking our plate away as soon as we had lifted the last forkful, still chewing, to pile on some more. For dessert, a plate of sweet latkes would be served (with raisins added), which we dipped in a bowl with cinnamon and sugar. After we had thanked her, she would say with an air of triumph: "And all that batter with only one egg." She was not without money, yet the shtetl lived within her, and she found it hard to spend money on herself. When she arrived at our house to spend the week with us kids, one of the first things out of her car would be a large cardboard box labeled BROKEN MIXED SWEET BISCUITS. Loose within the box were a variety of biscuits in various states of wholeness, biscuits that for one reason or another had failed whatever passed for quality control in the 1970s. These rejects would be loaded into boxes and sold in her local supermarket at knockdown prices, where my grandmother would get boxes and boxes of them.

Amid the chaos of family life, my grandmother would sit at our kitchen table and dip the biscuits serenely in her tea, although they were slightly stale, dusted with crumbs and sugar from other biscuits, and tasted of cardboard box. My coming downstairs in the evening barefoot in pajamas to nibble more biscuits (the box never seemed to empty) was one of the few things that would get her animated. "Look at you, coming down without your socks. You'll catch your death." Even at ten years old I knew that a cold was an infection that you caught from someone else, not something that you caught through your feet because you weren't wearing socks, but she was implacable. As far as she was concerned, catching a cold through your feet was an established fact, and exposure to the cold tile kitchen floor was reckless. She had similar views on the effects of sitting too close to the television (premature myopia), eating the crusts from bread (a cause of curly hair), and the medicinal effects of chicken soup.

My grandmother was a hundred and two when she died. She never considered that she was old, and in fact on one holiday was critical of the slippery hotel stairs because "old people might fall on them," entirely and unselfconsciously dissociating herself from the category. Her generation didn't talk about their feelings and didn't care much for displays of emotion. Throughout her whole life, she dissembled and obfuscated about her actual age so much that nobody knew how old she was. She made up one date of birth to give her doctor, a different one for social security, and a third at the hospital. She delighted in the fact that people seemed to believe her or complimented her on looking young for her age, even after she had already knocked a decade off. She waved aside the traditional telegram from the queen when she reached a hundred, saying vaguely that some error or other must have been made, so that I discovered her actual year and date of birth only when I went with my father to register her death.

For all of her slightly odd beliefs about health, she had an unshakable faith in doctors. She would dress up to see her GP, wearing her finest clothes. She would laugh respectfully at the doctor's jokes and quips and would do exactly as her doctor told her, even when what was prescribed was at odds with her own opinion. The doctor's word was non-negotiable. In short, her idiosyncratic beliefs about her health, about unstockinged feet—all of these were embedded in a rational framework, the belief that her doctor knew best. Her health beliefs were benign and endearing, yet she would never have talked out of turn at her doctor's surgery.

My observation of running clinics in my psychiatry service over the past eighteen years has been that now the doctor's opinion rarely goes unquestioned. Beyond the normal concerns anyone would have about their diagnosis, people's health beliefs have become more strident and dogmatic, and this has implications for the way healthcare is negotiated and delivered to patients. Increasingly patients come to my clinics telling me what diagnosis they are expecting me to give at the end of the consultation, a self-diagnosis that has already started to shape their lives and their interactions with society. They may already have joined a patient group of fellow sufferers and started to advocate for the diagnosis. Increasingly people come to my clinics believing they have autism spectrum disorders, bipolar disorders, adult ADHD (attention deficit hyperactivity disorders)—diagnoses that in former times would have been stigmatized and avoided. Those who don't do well in school may self-diagnose themselves with dyslexia. In my chronic fatigue clinic, patients often request a test for Lyme disease, believing that this is the cause of their illness. This is true even when they have never in their lives traveled to an area where the illness is endemic. I am always astonished by how many people remember having a target-shaped rash near the tick bite, a classic and highly specific sign of Lyme disease, only for the results of the test to be entirely normal.

Whereas in the past an individual who was supple and flexible would simply be good at yoga or gymnastics, now they come to clinics concerned about Ehlers-Danlos syndrome, which is a rare disorder that weakens the connective tissue in the body, rendering sufferers excessively flexible at the joints. In schools where there is a September 1 cutoff for the school year, the diagnosis of ADHD in childhood is greatly increased in the children born in August (the youngest in the class) compared with the children born in September (the oldest in the class). In other words, it is the child's immaturity relative to the rest of their classmates that is being conflated with a psychiatric diagnosis, rather than it being understood for what it is—namely a natural lack of maturity compared with their older peers.

What is it about our current culture that is driving this change, this rapid expansion of diagnoses? Well, for starters the medical profession must take a long hard look at itself and ask whether it serves the best interests of society to have an ever-expanding number of diagnoses, particularly where these diagnoses are very loosely defined. In its first incarnation in the 1950s, the American *Diagnostic and Statistical Manual of Mental Disorders* (*DSM-1*), which sought to cover all known mental illnesses, had 128 categories and was 132 pages long. In its current fifth overhaul, published in 2013, *DSM-5* has a total of 541 diagnostic categories and 947 pages. It seems that there are 413 further separate psychiatric illnesses identified over the past sixty years with which you can now suffer, something common sense tells you cannot be correct.

This allows normal human experience such as bereavement to creep into the diagnostic lexicon; bereavement depression was included for the first time in the most recent, fifth edition of the *DSM*. This is also true for the autism spectrum disorders, which seem to include an ever-increasing number of normal people into their sphere. The number of disorders you can be diagnosed with is steadily increasing, and the number of normal emotions or symptoms that can now be diagnosed as illness continues to expand. When every symptom or feeling can become a diagnosis, it reduces the individual's self-reliance and externalizes the responsibility for the individual's health or behavior. As a society, we are willing participants in this. People seem to want or need a diagnosis to explain or rationalize their behavior, even when their behavior is broadly within the boundaries of normal. Here a diagnosis can do real harm. It unnecessarily brings people into contact with the medical profession and renders them passive recipients of unnecessary medical interference. While patients may then feel that they are blameless for any symptom they display, the other side of the coin is that they believe themselves helpless, and this is very unhealthy. Whether this is the medical profession driving the individual's need to have every feeling and emotion validated by a diagnosis or whether medicine is merely reflecting the public mood, it is indisputably a substantial step in the wrong direction.

Aside from the steadily lengthening list of medical things that can go wrong with you, there is another reason why people are increasingly self-diagnosing: the misperception that diagnosing illness is easy and straightforward. We live increasingly in an age where experts are mistrusted. This mistrust has seeped into the public consciousness in the UK and more generally everywhere in the West; it is being fostered and encouraged by politicians. For politicians, of course, the reasons to mistrust experts are clear. The purpose is to downgrade inconvenient facts about their policies by casting doubt about any experts questioning the wisdom of them. A senior British politician, Michael Gove, famously said, "I think that the people of this country have had enough of experts . . . saying they know what is best and getting it consistently wrong." This statement caught the popular mood. Yet the logical consequence of this sentiment is that it allows for a free-for-all, in which anyone who holds an opinion believes it to be as valid as the next person's, whether they have any particular expertise or not. When it comes to medicine, the whole world of medical information available on the internet does not in itself make for an informed opinion. It takes a great deal of time, skill, and experience to make an accurate diagnosis. In his book *Thinking, Fast and Slow,* Daniel Kahneman may well have been correct when he said that "the accurate intuitions of experts are better explained by the effects of prolonged practice than by heuristics." Yet prolonged practice is indeed what all senior doctors have, which is why it is better to see a senior clinician than to have an amateur self-diagnose. I am reminded of the truism that if you think going to see a professional is expensive, you should try an amateur.

When it comes to self-diagnosis, a phenomenon known as the Dunning-Kruger effect becomes relevant. The Dunning-Kruger effect states that the less we know about something, the more we overestimate our ability to do it. Dunning and Kruger demonstrated that people who performed badly on tests of humor, logic, or grammar significantly overestimated their performance when asked how they thought they had done. Humans, it seems, just have a bias that overestimates their competence on things they know very little about. When we are ignorant, we think that doing an unfamiliar task will be pretty easy, and all it will take is a bit of practice or reading up on the internet to perform at the level of, say, a pilot or a psychiatrist. This is because people who know nothing do not even have enough knowledge to realize their own ineptitude. They don't know how much they don't know. But as people gain more experience and knowledge, they realize that their initial impressions of their abilities were vastly inflated and come to appreciate how much more knowledge and experience they need before they become competent. This was true in Kruger and Dunning's study, whereby improving skills of participants in the study led them to realize their limitations.

A few years ago, there was a UK government proposal for GPs to do "lumps and bumps" clinics. This was for minor skin blemishes, so that GPs, instead of referring patients to their local hospital for minor surgical procedures, could do the operation themselves at the GP practice, under local anesthetic. On the face of it, this made a good deal of sense. It would save patients from lengthy outpatient waiting lists and would free surgeons to do the bigger operations. This idea resonated with the general public. The proposal was followed by correspondence in the *Daily Telegraph* newspaper about the pros and cons of this new GP work. But one letter to the newspaper from an experienced surgeon blew the whole thing open. He pointed out that, from a technical point of view, minor operations to remove skin lumps were not that difficult and did not take long to learn. But what was much more difficult, indeed had taken him a lifetime of experience to learn, was knowing which skin lumps to leave alone.

It is consistent with the common experience that a little knowledge is a dangerous thing. Taking on an operation without fully realizing the pitfalls is foolish. I find that the less people know about something, the more certain they are about being right. And if you couple that with a general belief that anyone's opinion is just as valid as any other, it means that the dynamic of a consultation has shifted over the years. I now spend quite a lot of time at appointments discussing alternative diagnoses that the patient has brought. Some arguments have merit; many others are very farfetched. And from time to time, even when I am quite sure of a course of action to take, I can tell that my arguments have failed to convince a patient. Even when patients have been thoroughly investigated and discharged by the medical team, it can be hard for them to let go of the diagnosis that they brought in with them or to trust the expertise of doctors with decades of experience behind them. This can add months to their patient experience as they subject themselves to further referrals and investigations, before very often arriving back in my clinic.

At an individual level, self-diagnosis can turn a normal well person into someone preoccupied by their health and mistrustful of doctors. In addition, when people declare themselves to be ill, there is an impact on their family and work life that is far from benign. More worrying, though, is when a mistrust of experts and an overconfidence in individual ability to read the evidence combine to affect the wider public. This has been the cause for the dramatic decrease in administering vaccines such as the MMR, which has led to a public health crisis that could not have been imagined when measles was declared eliminated in the United States in 2000. In 2019, the CDC reported 1,282 cases of measles in thirty-one states, the highest number reported since 2000. In Europe, the picture is even worse, with what the World Health Organization referred to as "an alarming level" of cases, over 100,000 in a little over a year in Europe. And it should be remembered that measles is far from a benign disease. Before the measles vaccine was introduced in the 1960s, most children had measles in childhood. In the United States each year some 3 million to 4 million children were infected, of whom

48,000 were hospitalized, 1,000 developed encephalitis (a swelling of the brain), and 400 to 500 children died, according to CDC statistics.

A related issue is alternative medicine. Alternative health beliefs are part of a mindset that at one end of the spectrum is a benign and harmless addition to standard medical care, and at the other merges into overt conspiracy theory and paranoia. Generally speaking, doctors view the world of alternative health as a Wild West, a largely unregulated and incoherent system of healthcare delivery that can be dangerous, particularly when important clinical symptoms are misinterpreted. Even at its best, many alternative health conceptualizations of how the body works are at odds with accepted science. Illnesses are thought of in simplistic ways that fit the particular alternative medical theory rather than fit the evidence. They lack what is known as biological plausibility, the principle that an explanation for an illness needs to make sense to someone who understands the workings of a human body. Yet because their explanations of illness are simplistic, alternative health theories are easy to understand and therefore have a superficial appeal. Sometimes they appeal to common sense, in the way that it is common sense to think the earth is flat if you look as far as you can see along a sandy beach. We want life to be simple and understandable and to conform to a set of known rules that we can predict. This is what alternative health cures offer. It may be that your energies are poorly aligned or that you need a diluted bit of what made you ill in the first place. The websites selling treatments are replete with health information that looks like science. In fact they try to blind people with science, and to the lay observer, junk science can be hard to differentiate from the real thing. Sometimes the major selling point for alternative therapies is that they are "natural," but then of course so are ricin, tuberculosis, and anthrax.

When I ask patients if they are taking any over-the-counter or complementary remedies or dietary supplements, people usually look sheepish when telling me. They worry that doctors will see it as a rejection of their treatment, a reproach to their professionalism, and indeed some doctors do take it as such. Yet doctors should be interested in why people take alternative treatments. They need to be prepared to hear some uncomfortable answers, although few studies have looked in detail at this. One study showed an increase in more educated people, who find alternative treatments to be more consistent with their world view or philosophical attitudes toward health. Although in this study taking alternative treatments was not specifically taken as criticism of or dissatisfaction with conventional medical treatment, I couldn't help but wonder. In my experience, people are more likely to take alternative treatments for problems that they feel medicine does not address well. These include problems like dizziness, chronic pain, fatigue, and anxiety. These are the sort of nonspecific symptoms that modern Western medicine struggles to treat, and the sorts of consultations where patients come away from the doctor feeling irritated, not quite believed, not taken seriously, because rarely are these symptoms able to be packaged into a neat diagnosis and treatment plan. In deciding the parameters of what constitutes "real illness," medicine tends to ignore what is inconvenient—those illnesses that appear to lack an underlying biological basis. Symptoms like dizziness, which are hard to pin down, can be uncomfortably subjective for a scientific approach to diagnosis. Patients get if not exactly short shrift, then a shrug of the shoulders.

Doctors generally dislike admitting they have no idea how to account for a patient's presentation. Our training is focused on problem-solving, our self-esteem bound up with understanding and then fixing problems. Symptoms with no explanation, patients who won't get better, the lack of a treatment plan—all of these feel like failure. We all respond to failure in different ways, but it often ends up with blaming the patient, rather than honesty about the limits of our understanding of the human body. Perhaps their symptoms were not quite real. Maybe there's just something a bit off about them. Either way, patients quickly pick up on the change of tone and decide their problems may be better dealt with outside the usual medical settings.

By contrast, when patients describe their consultations with alternative health practitioners to me, what they focus on most of all is not the treatment they were given. The common theme is that the practitioner seemed to listen to them, have some time to spend with them, sympathize with them—all the things the doctors tend not to do when presented with vague and hard-to-treat complaints. And to a large extent, the treatment offered at the end by alternative health practitioners is beside the point. People go to alternative practitioners for the experience, the whole package, and not just the treatment. Yet the U.S. National Center for Health Statistics reported that Americans spend $30 billion a year on alternative health, and $12.8 billion on natural product supplements, which is a quarter of the amount spent on prescription drugs. This is surely telling a story of its own, that medicine is not providing something that people need or is not persuading them that the treatments that it offers are superior to other types of alternative medical practice.

I am often surprised by the lack of cynicism that is displayed toward the alternative healthcare industry, not by doctors but by the general public. The pharmaceutical industry is usually held up as nefarious, mercenary, and untrustworthy. Yet the alternative health industry seems to be even more shameless about its profiteering, with hardly a mention of this aspect of the industry. For sure, skepticism is expressed at the efficacy of the treatments, but somehow the industry as a whole is seen as naïve and misguided, rather than greedy and rapacious.

People mostly act in a rational fashion. They take health decisions guided by evidence, or allow themselves to be guided by professionals like doctors, whom people trust to assess the research evidence. Some people, like my grandmother, may hold a few slightly idiosyncratic but harmless health beliefs, although when it comes right down to it, they will back their doctor to get it right. Yet increasingly, in an age of consumer-driven healthcare, health beliefs have become more fragmented and less deferential. Medicine is not giving people what they need. I worry about what this means for the future of our profession and the health of the public.

MEDICAL MYSTERIES

I was on my way to work one morning, on the bus over London Bridge, when one of the hospital physicians called me. It was the first time we had ever spoken, and although our friendship has since blossomed over the years, this call was all business. He wanted to tell me about Gary, who was currently an inpatient on one of the medical wards, and to ask for my advice. Gary was a twenty-four-year-old man who had originally come to his family doctor the previous year complaining of abdominal pain, and on subsequent visits of light-headedness and fainting. His doctor had taken some blood tests, which all came back as normal, and sent a referral to the physician for a consultation in the outpatient department, which Gary did not attend.

Little was seen of him over the next several months, although there had been at least half a dozen attendances at different emergency departments in the intervening period. He would arrive at the emergency department sweaty, dizzy, and weak, and at the final two attendances, he'd had a seizure. Gary was admitted to the hospital after his seizures but discharged himself before investigations were completed, saying that he needed to get back to work.

This admission had come via the emergency department, too. Gary had complained of feeling light-headed and unwell, with ongoing abdominal pains, and of being unable to concentrate. On arrival at the hospital, alarmingly he had a seizure and lapsed into a coma. It was during this visit that a low blood sugar level was discovered. He was given intravenous glucose and quickly came round, then was admitted to the hospital for further investigations. Gary was suspected of having a rare type of tumor known as an insulinoma. These are tumors that produce insulin, the hormone responsible for lowering blood sugar levels. While not enough insulin leads to diabetes, tumors causing an excess of insulin lowers the blood sugar too far, leading to the range of problems that Gary exhibited.

Investigations proved frustrating. The usual blood tests did not seem to confirm the diagnosis. Yet the following evening Gary had another seizure, falling into a coma just as he had done days earlier, before once again being resuscitated with a glucose infusion. The medical team were starting to get worried and a little suspicious. Yet when the medical team challenged him, Gary denied having done anything that might have caused him such serious problems.

A few days later Gary again started to become sweaty and confused. By then a nurse had been assigned to keep a careful eye on him, and she quickly raised the alarm before noticing a packet of tablets among the tangled sheets on his bed. She saw immediately that the tablets were typically prescribed for diabetics, used to stimulate insulin production. How they had ended up with Gary was a mystery, but everything else began to make sense. Gary had been taking these tablets to deliberately lower his blood glucose levels, and in so doing had put his life in grave danger.

With overwhelming evidence now telling against him, Gary was again asked whether he might have done anything to cause his health problems. At first he maintained his insistence that he had not taken any tablets. Only later that day did he admit to the nurse what he had done. He had found the medication in his grandfather's bathroom cabinet while visiting him at his flat one day, and it was then that the idea came to him. He had slipped the tablets in his pocket, and thus began the series of events leading him to this point. The medical team had resolved one problem but now had another. They didn't know how they were going to be able to safely discharge him home.

Gary was in hospital pajamas sitting on a chair beside his bed when I came to see him. He seemed not the least bit chastened by the events of the preceding days, or if he was, it was certainly hard to tell. I asked him about his life. He spoke of an unhappy upbringing on a South London housing estate, which I happened to be familiar with. I had driven past it several times, a sprawling series of housing blocks in inner-city London. In fact I'd once been involved in a road traffic accident almost directly outside the block that Gary lived in. (I remember sitting on the low wall bordering the flats, stunned, rubbing the back of my neck, when a man leaned out of a third-floor window. "Hey!" he shouted in a heavy Jamaican accent. "Hey!" I turned to look up, wincing from the pain in my neck. "Hey! You!" he shouted. "You got whiplash!")

Gary's family background was complicated. His father had been in several relationships, both during and after his relationship with Gary's mother. The father was now back in Jamaica, and Gary had not seen him in years. He had two half brothers he knew about but was not close to; he couldn't remember the last time he had spoken to them.

After his father left, his mother had been in another relationship, to a man of whom Gary was terrified. He recounted to me how as a child when he heard his stepfather return home at night, almost always drunk, he would cower in his room, dreading what might happen. The slightest frustration would lead to a drunken rage. On one occasion, he recalled the smell of frying bacon reaching his room, then a banging of cupboards as his stepfather tried to locate the bread, which Gary had finished earlier that evening. He lay under his duvet, waiting for the inevitable beating. His mother never stuck up for him, finding it safer to side with her new partner than with her son, a position that Gary both understood and resented.

Gary struggled at school. He made few friends, telling me he did not take part in school life—no sports, music, or clubs—and just wanted to be left alone. At home, he longed to be cared for, but since that was never forthcoming, the next best thing was to be invisible. He never felt his life would amount to much and had few ambitions or ideas.

On leaving school, he tried to get work and had some part-time jobs on building sites, but steady work was interrupted by ill health. He began to experience abdominal pains and went back several times to his family doctor, who did not seem too concerned. Gary told me that it was then that he found the diabetic medication, and the idea came to him. He realized that it would likely give him real symptoms, and this would make his doctor take him more seriously. Once he started taking the tablets, though, he found it hard to stop.

He was hard put to explain what he wanted from his medical interactions. I asked him if it was to be cared for and looked after by the medical profession. This would be understandable, given a childhood of neglect. He shrugged his shoulders. He didn't seem to know himself why he did it. I queried if he realized how dangerous it was to take the medication, and I sensed Gary's engagement in the consultation start to waver.

He came back to my outpatient clinic on three more occasions over the following months, but I found it difficult to understand why. He played my questions with a dead hand. There was no flow to the consultations, which became a staccato series of questions and brief answers. Beyond the facts of his unhappy upbringing, he showed no curiosity in understanding why he behaved the way that he did. More worryingly, he had started to minimize what he had done, saying that people got low blood sugar all the time, and he didn't see it as too much of a problem. The brief window of opportunity that had opened up after his hospital admission was now closing, and I had been unable to take advantage of it. Soon Gary stopped coming to see me. I feared for his future. The most likely outcome was that he would continue to take the tablets and would play out this same scenario in other hospitals where he was not known, with all the risks that entailed. I never saw him again.

Whilst Gary's presentation was dramatic, evidence suggests that many other cases like Gary's, with more mundane presentations, go undiagnosed despite repeated attendances at their doctor. This is a function of how the medical profession is set up and operates. Doctors like to see themselves as detectives. Through a combination of skill, intuition, insight, and brave clinical decision-making, they like to be the ones to find the pathology and unlock the case that nobody else could make sense of. And then, perhaps by the administration of a little bit of this and a little bit of that, effect the treatment that nobody else could conceive of, lifting a lazy hand of acknowledgment to the grateful patient and awed colleagues. Many doctors dream of practicing what is jokingly called hero-based medicine, to differentiate it from evidence-based medicine. Yet this scenario, the fantasy propagated by *ER, House,* and all the other medical dramas, is vanishingly rare.

Evidence-based medicine (EBM) is the standard of modern-day practice. EBM means that we follow the best evidence available for the treatment of a particular condition, following protocols and guidelines that reflect the latest research. Where the research is thin, guidelines are added to by the opinion leaders, the great and the good in their particular field, who offer their wisdom as to best practice in the absence of clear evidence. EBM was promoted and popularized not to stop people from doing heroic things when the need arises but to stop maverick doctors from doing whatever it was that they wanted to. Mavericks in medicine are not uncommon. They are often well intentioned but usually dogmatic and misguided. They develop theories about disease and treatments unsupported by evidence and get cut adrift from sensible mainstream opinion. The worst of them see themselves as crusading visionaries, but in fact they are just not very good doctors. Even within the boundaries of normal good practice, I have seen over the years many doctors prescribe treatments to patients for which evidence is nonexistent, simply because they have a theory, or it is what their old boss used to do, or because they say they have "seen it work." That kind of attitude and practice should be discouraged. The history of medicine is full of treatments that should work, that we would like to think do work, but which are in fact hopeless.

A relatively recent example of this is treatment for back pain. When I was a medical student, the standard treatment for back pain was rest. It struck everyone as sensible and intuitive that the solution to a bad back was to lie in bed and not move around too much, until the back healed itself. This was held to be such a self-evident truth that it went entirely unchallenged and was probably not thought about much at all for decades—until research showed that this advice was worse than useless. In fact exactly the opposite approach is appropriate for most back pain. The research showed the importance of mobilizing yourself, of getting up and about as soon as practical, if you wanted the mechanical back problem to be resolved. As always, the research drew skepticism, then opposition, and is now taken as self-evident truth.

As EBM has developed, medicine has gradually become more homogenized, with practice standardized throughout many Western countries. Guidelines, consensus statements, and protocols have proliferated. On the one hand, this is a good thing. The quality of treatment a patient receives should be the same no matter which hospital they go to or where they live. It makes sense that treatments are standardized and based on good quality evidence, and that outcomes are reliable. Once a diagnosis is made, delivering evidence-based treatments is far preferable to the prejudices, idiosyncrasies, and erratic behavior of individual doctors. I have seen firsthand the damage done by some of these doctors in the patients referred to my clinic.

Yet EBM comes with downsides as well. One of the disadvantages is that the conformity that it promotes can stifle progress. Innovation tends to develop where local solutions can be developed to address local problems, because what works in one part of the country or in one hospital or with one particular group of patients may work less well in another. While research studies show outcomes in large groups of people, they may not always be best placed to highlight differences in subgroups of patients, or for a particular individual. And while following protocols should produce more reliable results, the studies on which they are based tend to be more idealized scenarios where diagnostic doubts or patients with other more complex problems have been excluded, so they are not always generalizable to the patient that you have in front of you in clinic. Furthermore, latitude in treating patients is how innovation develops. You want your doctor to know all of the rules and guidelines, but not always to follow them blindly.

But the biggest drawback of EBM is that reliance on guidelines can remove the need for critical thinking. Once you follow a guideline, you may find it easy to get drawn into the algorithm, starting with the first steps, and if they are not working, to follow the flow chart to the next step, with its steadily increasing doses and switches of medications, and finally to ever more esoteric combinations of medication. The problem is that much of the time, when we prescribe a medication, people do not take it and are reluctant to tell their doctor. In developed countries, according to a report for the World Health Organization, medication adherence (whether patients are taking medication as prescribed) among patients with long-term illness diseases averaged about 50 percent. In patients with depression, somewhere between 40 percent and 70 percent are taking their prescribed antidepressant treatment. In Australia, only 43 percent of the patients with asthma were taking their medication as prescribed all the time, and only 28 percent used their prescribed preventive medication. Doctors know this, the patients themselves clearly know this, but at an actual appointment, I don't think I have ever heard a patient spontaneously tell me they weren't taking their medication. Unless you ask, which doctors usually do not think to do, then guidelines are of little help.

When patients come back to the outpatient clinic and are no better, the commonest response is to increase the dosage of the medication because it is assumed that it is not working, rather than for the doctor to realize that the patient has not been taking it.

When I was a medical student, the chest doctor I was working for told me about a study he conducted in which he told asthmatic patients he was putting a microchip into their "preventer" inhaler, which they should be using twice a day. This was to see how regularly and accurately they were using their preventer inhaler, because the preventer is meant to avoid the need for the other inhaler, the reliever, meant to be taken only when the asthma is already worsening. What he found was that patients nearly always told him that they were using the preventer regularly, twice a day. They knew that the chip was recording this. What they did not know was the chip was also recording *when* the inhaler pump was activated, not just the number of times it had been activated. When he downloaded the data from the chip, he found that many people were pressing the pump repeatedly while they were in the waiting room before the appointment, to bring it up to the correct number of presses as if they had been taking it twice a day, as prescribed.

But the biggest criticism of guidelines is the "garbage in, garbage out" principle. You are not going to be able to put hamburger into a mixer and get steak out. So it is with guidelines. Guidelines can give you the greatest treatment algorithm in the world, but if you get the diagnosis wrong, then the starting point is the wrong one, and entering the guidelines just leads you further and further away from the correct destination.

The correct diagnosis can be more difficult to make than is generally acknowledged. In textbooks there is (obviously) the textbook example of a particular illness or disease. Yet this commonly does not accord with the real-world presentation of an illness, where the symptoms may be too early in their development to be apparent, or patients may emphasize particular symptoms they are worried about and ignore others, or the doctor may be more focused on a different disease, perhaps one they had recently missed in another patient. All of these can put a patient in the wrong treatment pathway. And there are other diagnoses, like Gary's, that can be unusual and difficult to understand, so that most doctors will not have made the diagnosis throughout their careers, despite it being commoner than is usually realized.

Gary's condition is known as factitious disorder and is thought to account for up to 1 percent of all inpatient hospital admissions, although my experience would suggest it is diagnosed far less commonly than that. In factitious disorder, the patient is deliberately causing the symptoms. For symptoms like pain, that is a relatively easy thing to do. For other symptoms, like blood in the urine, it takes a bit more thought from the patient. For example, when they are given the urine specimen pot, they will need to first produce the urine and then find a quiet place where they are unobserved before pricking their finger and adding a drop of blood to the sample in the pot. Nothing too dramatic is necessary, because the tests are very sensitive to microscopic amounts of blood, and it doesn't therefore need to be too obvious. Although factitious disorder is the name given to this kind of behavior, when extreme and persistent, it is usually referred to as Munchausen's syndrome.

The term "Munchausen's syndrome" comes from the fictional character Baron Munchausen, who was loosely based on a real person named Hieronymus von Münchhausen, an eighteenth-century German aristocrat who was known for recounting tall tales of his wartime exploits. The fictional character recounts the tales of his time as a solider and sportsman, telling impossible and unbelievable exploits, such as riding on a cannonball or pulling himself out of a swamp by his own bootstraps. In the book, the stories are told in a boastful way, and the baron appears to believe in his stories, no matter how implausible they are to a neutral observer. Yet in Munchausen's syndrome, the story may be entirely plausible, at least at first, and to the unwary can lead to medical disasters.

Why is it that doctors rarely, if ever, make this diagnosis? Well, for a start, doctors are usually pressed for time and generally take the patient's account of their problems at face value, since this is how we have been trained. As the great physician and "father of modern medicine" William Osler put it, "Listen to the patient. He is telling you the diagnosis." We tend not to consider that the patient may be actively misleading us. Undoubtedly another factor is that doctors do not enjoy the social awkwardness (let alone the extra time it takes) to challenge a patient's version of the events. It takes skill and patience, and even though we know that patients occasionally do deliberately simulate symptoms, which is to say they produce injuries to themselves to make it look like they are ill, or just make up the symptoms altogether, we rarely think it means the patient in front of us.

Why people do this is unclear. When I have asked patients, about half of them just deny it flat out, even when the medical evidence has proved beyond any doubt that their story is not medically possible. Of the patients who are able to acknowledge what they have done, only a small proportion engage meaningfully in treatment. I would add something else here. Although the whole Munchausen's label sounds vaguely comical and even quite jolly, with aristocratic Germans riding on cannonballs, the reality is very different. Several of the patients I have seen with this diagnosis have been among the most troubled I have seen during my career. Not in all of them, but in many of them, there is an undercurrent of something very dark and closed off in their personalities.

My first brush with this diagnosis was when I was a medical student. We had to shadow real doctors on call in the hospital, and I was in my surgical rotation. I had been extracted from the safety of the teaching hospital and cast in the real world of the understaffed but far friendlier district hospital. Surgery, I began to discover, was a lot less glamorous than was generally believed. My role as a medical student could be broadly subsumed under the term "dogsbody." I was learning mostly by observation, and the price for this opportunity was fetching, carrying, and generally being at the beck and call of the junior doctors, who in turn were abused to varying degrees by the senior registrar and consultant. And the surgical mindset, at least in those days, tended toward the rigid and unthinking.

It was a privilege accorded to medical students to assist in the operating theater, although the thrill very quickly wore off. The starting point was to be soundly, noisily, and very publicly dressed down by the scrub nurse, who would find any reason to fault your sterile technique in washing your hands or putting on the surgical gown and gloves. There's no scratching your nose or touching anything, once you're scrubbed up for theater. Yet once in the surgical gown, now boiling hot and still fizzing with embarrassment, I would feel my hot breath recirculating inside the surgical mask and itching trickles of sweat that I now couldn't wipe off, for fear of desterilizing my hands.

In the operating theater itself, after the initial excitement had worn off, the biggest problem then was boredom. As the operation slowly ticked along, with the surgeon by this stage a mixture of either high spirits (when it was proceeding well) or brittle, close-to-the-surface fury (when not), the atmosphere was never comfortable. While the moments of temper were stressful, the high spirits of a tyrant are no more relaxing, so generally the atmosphere was volatile. The final problem was cramping. I would usually be given a retractor to hold, to allow clearer vision to the surgeon by keeping the liver or loops of bowel or whatever out of the way of the surgical field. Maintaining this position eventually became uncomfortable, and I would swap hands, as you do with a heavy suitcase, trying hard not to let the bowel escape while in midswap. Sometimes I would daydream of last-minute goals in World Cup finals or the discovery of a lottery win, and on at least one such occasion was roused from my daydreams by the sharp rap of a surgical instrument on my knuckles, and looked down to discover the bowel had slipped under the retractor and was slowly sliding back into the abdominal cavity.

It was during this student placement that a man was admitted to the surgical ward. He complained of abdominal pain, and even as a student, I thought his story didn't really feel right, although the surgeons, busier and seemingly interested only in the hard facts rather than the nuances of the story, seemed happy to accept it at face value. He had a history of repeated surgeries, all carried out abroad (conveniently so, I felt), so it was impossible to check up on the facts. His usual work, he said, was on board a ship, now at sea, so that there was nobody around to corroborate his account of his health problems. Inevitably, there were no family or friends to talk to. His abdomen was a crisscross of scars, and his explanations for them varied. Eventually, he was taken to the operating theater for a laparotomy, an operation in which the abdomen is opened up for the surgeon to have a good look around, in an attempt to discover the cause of his intense abdominal pain.

He was back on the ward a couple of hours later, the surgeons none the wiser despite their diagnostic operation. The patient himself continued his evasions and inconsistencies about his previous medical history, his personal details, or any potentially useful diagnostic information, even as he lay in bed recovering from his operation. He even sent the team on a wild-goose chase, suddenly "remembering" he might have medical records from a hospital that he had been to in London "somewhere near a station." Of course that was no sort of clue, as most London hospitals are located by a railway station, but naming all of the hospitals close to a station failed to ring a bell with him. One evening, he slipped away from the ward, never to return. In all likelihood, as is the nature of factitious disorder, he would reenact the same scenario at another hospital a few weeks later.

Factitious disorders occupy a gray hinterland in medicine. While the patients themselves know that they are deliberately simulating their symptoms, it is not the same as malingering, where the individual knows exactly why they are pretending to be ill. People malingering do so for a clear gain, such as claiming sickness benefits or defrauding insurers, and they are fully aware of why they are doing it. Patients with factitious disorder also deliberately fake their symptoms, yet the reasons they do so are less clear, not only to the doctor but also to the patients themselves. Various theories have been advanced to explain such strange behavior that could account for why individuals readily submit themselves to unnecessary, painful, or even dangerous investigations and operations. It is usually thought to be a desire to inhabit the "sick role."

The sick role was described in 1951 by the American sociologist Talcott Parsons and is generally thought of as a social contract. In this social contract, an individual feeling unwell submits himself for examination by a doctor, who will legitimize his suffering by making a diagnosis and excuse the individual from his normal social responsibilities, such as going to work. In return, the individual must want to get better, by following the doctor's advice, so that he can return to his normal role in society. The interval from when a doctor makes a diagnosis until the individual is declared better is the period in which the person inhabits the sick role. It is thought to be this role that an individual with factitious disorder wishes to perpetually inhabit, remaining within the care of the medical profession. While disordered personalities are usually suggested as a cause, this is in itself rather too nonspecific as a diagnosis, and not particularly helpful either in treating individuals.

My second experience of factitious disorder came one February night. At this point I had been a doctor for just over twelve months and had applied to work in the Accident and Emergency department, to gain a bit of real experience and try to feel like a proper doctor. The first year of being a doctor is closely supervised. After that, the level of supervision was pretty hit or miss, and working in the emergency department was far more miss than hit. At nights, I was the only doctor, so between nine P.M. and nine the next morning I bluffed and sweated and tried my best not to make too much of a mess of things. It seems absurd now that this could happen—that a junior doctor barely out of medical school could be the most senior person in the whole department—but that's just how it was back then. Often, during the quiet moments in the department, the nurses and I would sit down together and play Guess the Diagnosis.

The game was that you had to guess the patient's diagnosis by observing the way they checked themselves in at reception, which you could observe from the CCTV screen in the corner of the room. Urinary retention was fairly easy to spot, even on a grainy CCTV image, with the patient more or less doubled over and sweaty. I recall a large Scotsman who had drunk six pints, then discovered once he got home that he could not urinate. As the pressure built up, still drunk and filled with catastrophic thoughts of his bladder exploding, he realized he wasn't going to be able to sleep it off and finally came in at about six A.M. When I catheterized him, the relief was immense. He looked up at me with such a profound sense of relief and peace of mind, smiling tiredly, and with a lovely Scottish burr said, "I feel like I've been blessed, Doctor," and more or less immediately fell into a deep and satisfied sleep. I wrote an outpatient referral to the urology team and carried on with my shift.

Through the CCTV you would see checking in at reception the assorted punch fractures, toothaches (we never learned a thing about those at medical school), lacerations, drunkenness, psychotic breakdowns, bad trips, asthma, heart attacks, chest infections, wobbly geriatrics, strokes, local homeless trying to keep warm, smoke inhalation, and my personal favorite—the Sunday-morning bagel clinic. In the North London neighborhood where the emergency department was located, with a large Jewish population of people, bagels were a staple of Sunday-morning brunch. And every Sunday, we ran the "bagel clinic," an injury caused when the patient held the bagel they were slicing in half in one hand, the knife in the other, then would cut through the bagel, out the other side, and lacerate the palm of their hand.

I was once again playing Guess the Diagnosis during my night in casualty when I saw a man on the CCTV screen entering the department, holding his arm. This time the diagnosis was less clear. A fracture? Dog bite? Dislocation? It turned out to be the latter, a dislocated shoulder. First, you must take an X-ray to confirm the shoulder is dislocated. Then you reduce the shoulder (which means putting it back in place) by (here my memory gets hazy) administering large quantities of powerful painkillers and muscle relaxants, getting the patient to drape his arm over the back of the chair, and pulling hard. The shoulder goes back into place with a satisfying clunk, and it is one of the very few moments when you get to feel like a real doctor. Instant cure.

The patient in this case didn't want an X-ray beforehand. This was unusual, and being a somewhat fastidious doctor, I objected. But somehow, and to this day I don't quite know how, the patient talked me out of it. Looking back, I see it as some sort of witchcraft. He said he had several dislocations before and so knew the symptoms. He said I must be a rugby player, which he could tell by looking at me, so I should have no problem reducing his shoulder. At this point, I temporarily forgot that I barely register five feet seven and had never before (and twenty-five years later, as it turns out, never since) been complimented on my physique.

The drugs were administered. The patient looked woozy, and I hung his arm off the back of the chair. I pulled with steady traction. Nothing. I kept up the steady traction, sweat now forming on the top of my brow. Still nothing. I just couldn't do it. I could feel the nurse's gaze on me, wondering if junior doctors were getting less competent or whether it was just me.

I stopped what I was doing, stood up, and took stock. A story came to mind that I'd once heard about Houdini, the famous escapologist, told by a rabbi (also, coincidentally, a psychiatrist) in the United States called Abraham Twerski. The story goes that Houdini was offered a challenge to get out of a locked room. The door was slammed closed, and Houdini got to work. He was there for half an hour trying to un-pick the lock, regurgitate keys, or whatever it was that Houdini did, yet every technique he tried failed. Houdini had finally been defeated! Eventually, he slumped down exhausted. And as he slumped down, he knocked the door handle down. The door swung open. And the lesson was: even the great Houdini can't unlock a door that hasn't been locked in the first place.

As the realization dawned, it all started to make sense. The shoulder couldn't be reduced because it was never dislocated in the first place! That was why the patient hadn't wanted me to X-ray it. I went back to the patient, this time with an X-ray form and a list of questions, but the patient got up, the effects of the sedative drugs still evident, and stood shaking on his legs for a few moments like a newborn foal before making his way unsteadily into the cold London night.

I stood there bewildered for a few minutes. What on earth was going on? Here was a man in perfectly good health who was pretending to be ill. He was going to submit himself to a painful procedure, with sedating medication (itself not without risk), carried out by a new doctor in the middle of the night, for no health benefit whatsoever.

Again I thought back to my medical student sociology and the chapter in my book entitled "The Doctor-Patient Relationship." I thought back to the doctor-patient "contract," the sick role, and the way that this is taught in medical school as a concrete set of rules governing all doctor-patient behavior. The real world, as I was discovering, was far messier than that; indeed, it was swimming in uncertainty. The patient who had just left the department was undoubtedly unwell, but just not in the way that it had first appeared. Although his presentation was with a physical complaint, the only treatment that he needed was psychiatric.

Over the years, I have seen many patients fox doctors for weeks, sometimes even months or years, with unexplained physical symptoms. Endless rounds of tests and investigations are carried out and fail to explain the problem. The patient remains ill, and the expense to the NHS of the unnecessary investigations is huge. Doctors generally fear missing a diagnosis, so patients who want to deceive doctors, usually for complicated motives that relate to their personalities and their often-unhappy background, can therefore string doctors along. Eventually, if the patient persuades the doctor to perform surgery, they can end up with very real problems, too, a consequence of their surgery, just to complicate things. I have seen patients with normal kidneys removed, patients who have deliberately falsified blood test results, patients who have caused strange skin rashes or have injected joints to cause infection—and the real treatment all these patients need is to see a psychiatrist, although they rarely do. Few psychiatrists have an interest and expertise in this specialized area of medicine, and this itself reflects the funding priorities of healthcare systems. The problem of funding is compounded by the fact that patients with these kinds of problems usually remain invisible in healthcare settings. Doctors rarely recognize it, and patients are unresisting, encouraging even, of the invasive investigations and treatments they are being given.

All this is because we have largely believed what we have been taught in the textbooks and at medical school. We believe that medicine is a science, and that patients coming for our help do so because they want us to delineate the pathology, the bit of the body gone wrong, the underlying cause of their troubles, so that we can treat it and effect the cure. This is the cool, rational, scientific approach to disease we have convinced ourselves that medicine is. We have forgotten that patients come to doctors for all sorts of reasons, many of which are unconnected with health. Many people presenting as patients have no interest in getting better, in the sense of giving up their symptoms—the symptoms themselves gain them access to the medical profession. Indeed, they want to remain within the embrace of the caring professions, and that is the goal in itself. Getting better means recognizing and then healing the psychiatric pain that they have been in, rather than repeatedly investigating their symptoms. That this illness is mostly unrecognized when it presents to doctors says something about how doctors are trained to think. Sad to say, medicine is a long way behind on dealing with patients like this.

MEANING

"My mind to your mind. Your thoughts to my thoughts." Mr. Spock, a character from *Star Trek*, was performing a "mind meld." It allowed him to access the thoughts of the person with whom he was telepathically connected, and as I watched the episode, it occurred to me that Spock would make a very efficient psychiatrist. Psychiatry is conducted at the level of the mind, and the purpose of the psychiatric consultation is to access the mental experiences of the person being interviewed.

We do this by careful observation and close questioning. Rather than being a free-associating, go-where-the-conversation-takes-us chat, a psychiatric history is a semi-structured interview, in which certain ground has to be covered. I always begin with the presenting complaint, which is the reason the patient has been referred to see me. It might have been a long time in the making, so this can sometimes take twenty to thirty minutes of listening, probing, and clarifying. You then need to know the patient's past medical and psychiatric history, as these can have a bearing on a diagnosis. Time is also spent covering family and personal history, sometimes itself a muddled and lengthy story, as well as covering use of alcohol and drugs.

When this is done well, there is a real skill to it. It comes from having time, experience, expertise, and the ability to understand what is being said, as well as to hear what is not being said. It requires an understanding of mental illness and human nature.

When I listen to a patient, I am making assumptions the whole time, only some of which turn out to be true. I may wonder why someone with a stable family background and middle-class parents has been unable to hold down a job for more than a few months at a time. What does that say about them and their ability to get along with people? Why did they never make friends at school? What made their home life so bad? Are they hinting at abusive relationships? Or why at the age of thirty-five have they never had a relationship that lasted more than a few weeks? We can all be unlucky, but it could be that this says something about a patient's self-esteem and confidence, or about a more profound inability to progress beyond superficial relationships into something deeper, that reflects their underlying personality structure.

I also take note of nonverbal cues. I can't remember who it was who said that all behavior is communication, but it's true—we communicate with one another through everything we do, from the way we style our hair to our posture and the clothes we wear. We don't realize it, but things like eye contact, fidgety behavior, tone of voice, the amount someone talks, and reactions to questions are all saying something. Tattoos are another expression of who someone is. Someone with STAY STRONG in large Gothic script down their arm would have it only because they feel weak or vulnerable and want to encourage themselves.

Noticing these things, in my case at least, is not a deliberate process; my impression of someone is instantaneous. Social class, occupation, marital status, personality, and likely diagnosis—all these things seem to come to me in the blink of an eye. I have developed a fairly reliable instinct over the years. This is from observing people, talking in detail to them, and building up patterns of behavior and interactions. It is not magic, nor is it infallible, and all these impressions need to be backed up in a thorough interview.

This ability to make a judgment about character is unique not only to psychiatrists, but to anyone whose job it is to observe human behavior. Airport security is a case in point. During the 9/11 attacks in the United States, airline staff were concerned enough about the behavior of the terrorists coming through Newark airport that they retained their boarding passes, rather than discard them as they usually would have. The airline employees formed an instant impression that these passengers were different from others. Based on their vast experience of passengers boarding planes, they felt that something was different, something just didn't sit right with them, even if at that stage they could not quite put their finger on what it was and could never have guessed at the catastrophe about to unfold.

If all this makes a psychiatric interview sound rather intense and unpleasant, I would also note that the most common thing that patients say to me after I have seen them is that they have enjoyed the experience. I think this is for two reasons: because people like talking about themselves to someone who is properly listening, and because they are relieved that they have come through unscathed from an experience that they were dreading. People used to worry that if they said the wrong thing, they'd end up getting sectioned—involuntarily committed to the hospital—but I hear that less now. The truth is that they'd have to say something pretty desperate for the thought to even enter my mind.

I'm often asked if I can tell whether someone is lying to me. People have all sorts of reasons for lying. Some are financial—for example, to gain compensation in a clinical negligence claim. Some people lie to doctors so they can be looked after and investigated or so they can co-opt a relative into continuing as a carer. Other people lie out of embarrassment, for fear of having to admit a fight they got into, a nasty comment they made, or the abuse they're suffering. In short, people lie for all sorts of reasons, some of which are defensive, while others are designed to deceive and manipulate. I remember one man making a preposterous claim about a surgical procedure having gone wrong and an instrument being left in his body; he was suing the hospital, though I knew his claim was anatomically impossible. Inevitably, the press had got involved and wrote an outraged TOP DOCS MESS UP sort of headline.

Another colleague, while writing a medicolegal report, told me about a claimant who had been left disabled by a road traffic accident that had occurred some years before. My colleague had written a very sympathetic report after conducting a lengthy clinical interview and a thorough review of the notes. It was just as she was putting the finishing touches to the report that she received a DVD of the claimant from the insurance company, who had employed someone to covertly follow and film him. The footage showed the claimant at the train station on his way to the interview, skipping lightly up the steps and up to the ticket barrier, before unfolding his walking aids and effortfully walking the remaining hundred yards to the office. The same happened after the interview: a labored and slow walk to the station, after which the walking aids were folded into his bag and he trotted normally down the stairs to the platform.

I can think of occasions when my initial impressions of a patient have left me entirely wrong-footed. It is disconcerting. For a moment the aura of confidence that every good clinician needs to project can crack. I think back to the patient whom I treated for depression, only to belatedly discover that heavy cocaine use was in fact the cause of all his ills, and which retrospectively explained my failure to make any headway whatsoever in his treatment. Eating disorders are another commonly missed reason for things that just don't add up, and again I think back to the times when I got wise to this behavior only months into treatment. The danger is that once your mind is made up about the patient in front of you, it's easy to stop noticing your biases. Evidence that contradicts your initial impressions is minimized or ignored, and only when the lack of progress is obvious and the sense of unease builds does a rethink become unavoidable. I carry around with me several of these cases, their names and diagnoses etched into my brain as a reminder of the effects of hubris. I've been handed a few lessons along the path of my career. It makes me wince to think of them, but there's only one appropriate reaction to being taught a lesson in life—learn it well. Being an experienced consultant has made me more circumspect, more aware of the fallibilities of human judgment, more flexible in my thinking.

The one sure piece of advice I can offer is that it's really difficult to tell if someone is lying to you, and almost impossible to spot when you're lying to yourself. Trying to weed out the lies from the truth in a consultation is more a feeling than a science. Sigmund Freud talked about "chattering fingertips" giving the liar away, which seems to have slipped into the popular consciousness, but that's a load of twaddle. As Andrew Malleson writes in his marvelous book *Whiplash and Other Useful Illnesses*, Freud was a good psychotherapist but would have made a lousy customs officer—there's no real "tell" for a liar. The only thing that helps me judge whether someone is lying to me is my experience. For example, when someone gets the simple, obvious questions wrong, stumbling and hesitating when I ask them how old they are, it makes me sit up. When people want to tell a big lie, they use a lot of their mental resources trying to remember all the details of it, in order not to give themselves away. The lie is being mentally rehearsed, so it is the small, unexpected questions that knock them off script and lead to a stumble.

Even when patients are not trying to deceive you, it is not always easy to understand what is really driving their emotions. I remember doing my psychiatry attachment as a medical student and being asked by the consultant psychiatrist to see a twenty-year-old Welshwoman, who had been referred because she was depressed and not responding to treatment. I spent an hour with the patient as she told me a long and involved story about her depression, which had begun after the death of her uncle. She told me that he had been murdered by her boyfriend, who was now in prison, but her depression didn't quite add up—the symptoms were vague and a little inconsistent. I took the rest of her history, but there wasn't much that was out of the ordinary: some alcohol, some minor drug use, a series of casual jobs, and some minor fraudulent activities to pay for the things in life that she couldn't afford. It wasn't entirely hanging together, but then again, her uncle, to whom she had been close, had died under very tragic circumstances, which I thought was probably enough to precipitate the depression.

I presented my findings to my consultant in his office, with the patient also present. The consultant is the senior doctor in the team, who takes overall responsibility for the care of any patient seen by one of his or her junior doctors. For a medical student, every case would need to be screened. Presenting patients' histories to the consultant was a good opportunity to learn how an experienced doctor would manage cases and was all part of the apprenticeship. The consultant listened to me and said little, before asking the patient a few supplementary questions about the murder of her uncle. She told him how her boyfriend had stabbed her uncle and been sent down for life.

"But you still love your boyfriend," he said gently, a statement rather than a question. I held my breath. It seemed an outrageous assertion and I wasn't sure how she was going to react, but I've never forgotten what happened next. I had always thought the expression "bursting into tears" was a cliché, because until that moment I had never seen someone actually burst into tears. It was a sudden thunderclap of emotion, shocking and dramatic. Everything that I had failed to get out of the patient in an hour-long conversation had been elicited in minutes. The terrible guilt, anguish, and misery of loving both your uncle and the man who had murdered him had been weighing her down but now burst through.

That case illustrated to me the constrained way of thinking I was developing. I had decided that depression was the diagnosis and had asked questions that supported this theory. Yet psychiatry is not simply about trying to make a psychiatric diagnosis. It is about understanding the limits of a diagnosis. Sometimes a diagnosis just doesn't really capture the problem, and then it becomes a catchall that stifles further thought. It limits rather than enlightens. The diagnosis of depression is a good example of where the range of human experience can easily be cast aside in favor of a reflex that assumes that all unhappiness must be attributed to depression.

When I met Rose for the first time, we were in my upstairs clinic room, the one with the window looking directly out at a brick wall. Fire regulations meant that patients had to go through a series of doors to get into the room. There's not enough room to open the second door to the clinic when you've opened the first door from the main staircase; you are forced to wait in a dark, narrow corridor for the first door to close, which it does slowly on a hydraulic hinge, before you can open the second. Sometimes I end up in uncomfortably close proximity to a patient as we try to make small talk while willing the first door to close so we can open the second.

Once we were settled in the clinic room, I started to take Rose's history. She seemed straightforward enough; in fact, she looked slightly defeated. She was casually dressed in velour jogging bottoms and a sweatshirt, the type of clothes that don't need ironing. I guessed she was over forty, although she told me she was thirty-six. Her face looked pasty and drawn; she seemed to have food stuck to her cheek, and I wondered whether she had stopped taking care of herself. Rose had grown up in South London before leaving school at sixteen and getting pregnant at seventeen. She had an uneasy relationship with her family. She had been quite bright at school but was never encouraged to work hard, so she left with a few mediocre qualifications and no career aspirations. She didn't really participate in school life, and from the picture she painted, it wasn't really that sort of school. After the birth of her baby, her partner admitted to an affair, which she had pretended not to notice during her pregnancy, and the relationship ended. Her parents helped out with childcare, but a few years later she got pregnant again, by a man who abused her. She said he was so angry to discover she was pregnant that on one occasion he had thrown her down the stairs.

She was now single and hadn't been in a relationship for five years. Her elder child was grown up and had left home, and her younger daughter was fifteen and didn't involve Rose in her life. Rose had no job, little money, and nothing to do. She told me she was consistently sad, withdrawn, hopeless, and lacking in motivation. She had been on different courses of antidepressants over many years ("I've tried them all") with no particular benefit. I wasn't sure what she thought might be different this time, but I took her history and began to understand her sense of despair. In the street outside the office, some drilling started. I looked out the window and watched a car drive slowly down the road and turn left. I realized that neither of us had said anything for thirty seconds.

On paper, this looked like depression. Rose had all the features of the illness: sadness, hopelessness, helplessness, pessimism, and an inability to enjoy life. Yet it didn't feel like depression when I spoke to her. I began to think of Viktor Frankl's *Man's Search for Meaning,* a superb book written in the concentration camps of World War II. In a moving account of what it was like to live in that environment, Frankl explains that when all sense of meaning is extinguished from life, living becomes intolerable. He explains that we fundamentally crave a sense of purpose in our lives; if we understand the why, we can withstand the how. When we have a purpose in life, we can keep going despite our suffering. But when we lack a sense of purpose, our suffering becomes meaningless and impossible to withstand.

I have seen many depressed patients for whom multiple courses of antidepressants have failed to make any difference, and who come to me labeled as "difficult to treat" or as having "treatment-resistant depression." And in nearly all cases, they have not got depression at all, but a life that lacks any higher goals. Their actions are meaningless and the days drift by—who wouldn't feel sad, hopeless, pessimistic, and unhappy under those circumstances? Frankl talked of our nihilism not as a belief in nothing but as a belief in "nothing but." If we are "nothing but" intelligent apes, "nothing but" a machine, then living becomes futile. We need to believe that what we do matters, that it transcends our own immediate needs. Mahatma Gandhi intuitively understood how meaning is achieved in life when he said, "The best way to find yourself is to lose yourself in the service of others."

I once read an article in *The New York Times* about Japanese labor laws. In Japan, firing employees is difficult. For employees who refuse a redundancy package, companies respond by not giving the employee any work. Day after day, employees have to come to work and sit there idly, unwanted and unproductive. Every day they achieve nothing. The phone would never ring for them, their ideas would not be listened to—in fact, their very presence at work would be an exercise in sheer pointlessness. It would be utterly demoralizing, a kind of living death. The humiliation and shame and futility of that daily existence would not come close to compensating for the salary. I know that I would be out like a shot.

I wondered if Rose was experiencing something of this sort, feeling a lack of meaning in her life. I expect most people from time to time ask themselves whether their actions in life serve any useful goal. Perhaps they might also ask themselves whether there is more to life than fashion, pleasure, drinking, cars, yachts, and holidays. All these things do, of course, provide transient pleasure, but they don't give a sense of deep and lasting happiness. Without a meaningful role, you are not usually fulfilled or happy.

I asked Rose when she had last been really happy. She thought for a moment before telling me about a time when she took her niece to Heathrow Airport. It wasn't an occasion that many of us would think of as fulfilling, but to Rose it confirmed that she still served a useful purpose in life, so it gave her a sense of satisfaction.

I developed a treatment plan for Rose based on the idea of finding purpose, one that didn't rely on antidepressants. We looked at the things she had been good at and had enjoyed and tried to find ways in which she could volunteer, perhaps building up her skills to gain employment. It turned out that one of the things she had always enjoyed was cycling. She had an old bike she didn't use much, but she began to cycle more and enjoyed getting out of the city. When she got an interview for a part-time job at a local bike shop, I think I was as nervous as she was. It didn't seem appropriate to ask her to let me know how it had gone, so I waited for her next appointment.

A couple of months later, Rose was back. She had gotten the job in the bicycle shop and felt better than she had for many years. She was still on income support but felt a great deal better about herself, and the issue of antidepressants felt less pressing. She shyly mentioned that she had started dating one of her colleagues, and she was clearly relishing her sense of normality. Over the next few months, her life gradually started to develop a structure, and by the time I discharged her, she had been hired full time and was engaged to be married.

I remember Rose because cases rarely go that way. There are usually many reasons why a patient feels stuck and helpless, and any suggestion is met with a range of counters. A typical conversation might go like this:

"Is there some daytime activity that you might enjoy?"

"I have to pick up my child from school."

"Perhaps there are some after-school clubs your daughter could go to?"

"She doesn't like them."

"Well, maybe you have relatives or friends who could pick her up a few days a week?"

"No, she wouldn't like that."

"Could you perhaps look for something part-time in the mornings after dropping her off?"

"There isn't anything like that."

"So you mean it's not even worth looking?"

Although the answers sound plausible, they tend to amount to the fact that the patient is embedded in a cycle of helplessness, and the unwary clinician can end up being drawn into this if he or she is not careful. After feeling like a victim of circumstance for such a long time, people generally respond with the personality of victimhood, which usually means that they become helpless and attribute blame to other people, institutions, depression, bad luck, or poor timing, and ignore any notion of their own ability to change things. It can take time, patience, and skill to bring the patient around to your way of seeing things, but the alternative is to keep prescribing antidepressants that you know deep down won't work, to treat a diagnosis of depression that you don't believe in. While it is undoubtedly harder to help people frame their problems as a deficit of meaning in their life rather than a deficit of serotonin in their brain, having the experience and confidence to be able to do this can make all the difference in the world.

ACCEPTANCE

When I first saw Marianne, sitting in a chair by her hospital bed, I had to suppress my shock. I had heard about her from a junior doctor, who had presented her case in our weekly team meeting before our ward round. A forty-two-year-old woman, she had spent three months in the hospital some years before, as a result of severe bowel disease. She had now been admitted to the ward because of her weight, which had been declining significantly. Initially, and understandably, this was thought to be a result of a recurrence of her inflammatory bowel disease, yet she had been investigated and nothing had come to light. Eventually, with her weight dangerously low, she was admitted to the hospital, in an attempt to uncover the problem and feed her, so as to reverse her weight loss. She felt too nauseated to eat, so a feeding tube was inserted up her nose and down her esophagus into her stomach, with nutrients delivered through bottles connected to the tube. Unfortunately, the tube kept coming out, mostly at night when she would catch it on something as she slept, so her weight continued to drop.

As is common for the referrals to psychiatry in a general hospital, she had been seen by several different departments before us. Gastroenterology had investigated her bowel function and had looked into whether her weight loss was being caused by poor absorption of food. Other teams looked for a possible cancer to explain her weight loss. Scopes, probes, X-rays, and scans had all been done, but the medical team were no nearer to understanding her weight loss. She had been in the hospital for nearly two weeks by the time the admitting team wondered whether psychiatry might be able to help solve this puzzling case.

After the team meeting, as we made our way from our team base to the ward where Marianne was wasting away, I wondered whether psychiatry would have anything to add to her care. I always find it useful to think through the diagnostic possibilities before I meet a patient, and as we walked, I speculated about what we might find. It crossed my mind that the physicians might have missed something that they would later kick themselves for, yet I knew them as meticulous and careful clinicians, so this seemed unlikely. But how might I account for a non-physical cause? I had seen depressed patients stop eating and lose weight as a result before, but rarely to this degree. And surely it would be hard for the nurses, doctors, physiotherapists, and other staff who routinely care for patients in a hospital not to have noticed that a patient was too depressed to eat. In my experience of such cases, patients who are this depressed speak very little, and in a slow, monotonous tone. Their bowed posture and dejected demeanor would surely have been obvious to everyone, so depression seemed improbable as a cause of weight loss.

I wondered whether illicit drug use might have been responsible; it is often an explanation for things that can't be explained otherwise. Serious drug use has a variety of unpredictable physical health consequences. Inpatients using drugs can be quite inventive in the ways they bring drugs into the hospital, and hospital staff rarely suspect patients of drug use. Within the "rules" of a normal doctor-patient relationship, good faith is assumed on both sides. It can be hard to practice medicine if you are constantly suspicious that a patient is trying to hoodwink you, or to be a patient if you suspect that your doctor might be taking bribes to prescribe a certain medication.

I am not particularly cynical, yet like most doctors who have been practicing for some years, I have been tripped up by being too trusting and have learned to question what people tell me. A few years ago, nurses suspected a patient of misusing alcohol, but his angry denials and hurt at my suggestion dissuaded me from asking any more questions for fear of causing him offense. He was an articulate middle-aged man, and I remember him complaining that drink was all in the past, but still nobody would trust him. In any case, he said, he hadn't left the ward, so where could he be getting alcohol from? This question was answered some days later, when I discovered that he had a vodka-filled hot-water bottle that nobody had thought to check. I supposed that illicit drug use was a possibility for Marianne, although I still thought it was unlikely that this would have gone unnoticed.

I arrived at the ward, found Marianne's bed, and introduced myself. She motioned to a chair by her bed and I perched on it awkwardly, with the rest of my team standing behind me. Propped up in bed and skeletally thin, Marianne was wearing just a nightie, with the bedsheets in a tangle toward the foot of her bed. The first thing I saw were her knees, which seemed huge compared to her thighs. Her head looked like a moon perched on tiny shoulders. I glanced around the bedside, something that I do instinctively, because you can learn a great deal about a person from the items they choose to surround themselves with. There was none of the paraphernalia that most people accumulate after a couple of weeks in hospital. Where were the cards, family photos, puzzle books, newspapers, novels, bottles of energy drink, packets of biscuits, and bowls of fruit?

Marianne spoke about her health problems in a rather mechanical way. She seemed puzzled by her sustained weight loss and spoke about how frightened she was of what might be causing it. Her speech seemed somehow rehearsed, as if it lacked any emotional depth, so I changed tack and asked a little about her background.

She had been born into a family of high achievers. Her parents were both investment bankers, and her sister had studied at Oxford before a successful career in one of the big law firms. Marianne, by contrast, had always believed that she was falling short and was living in her sister's shadow. She felt that whatever she did was never good enough and described the atmosphere while she was growing up as cold. She had been given everything she wanted except for the love and admiration she craved most. Her parents were practical and efficient rather than warm and caring; she felt starved of praise or attention. As she spoke, tears rolled down her cheeks. The memory of these feelings of rejection and inadequacy was still raw, and she seemed lost in her own world. "Not good enough," she said quietly, though not in response to any question.

Marianne had taken a job as a bookkeeper after leaving school, and although she had a few brief relationships, she had never married. Her self-esteem was low; she saw herself as ugly and unlovable. In an attempt to regain a sense of control and to feel better about herself, she began to restrict her eating, believing that she would gain the admiration and respect of other people if she was thin.

As I think back to that conversation, it is the tears that I remember most clearly. Once we began a deeper discussion after the initial small talk at the start of the consultation, her tears switched on like a tap. This was the first time she had admitted to anyone that she had been deliberately starving herself. She wanted to look better, to feel noticed and loved; she hoped people would admire her self-control. She admitted to removing the feeding tubes at night; they hadn't caught on things and come out on their own. She had always felt that if she was just a couple of pounds lighter, then she would be fulfilled and self-confident, but she now realized that she was losing control of the situation. I asked her whether she thought she was now too thin. There was a pause, and she said that she wasn't sure, although she was aware of the medical team's concern. Out of curiosity, I asked her to draw what she thought she looked like—I had read a study suggesting that women with eating disorders had a distorted view of their own bodies that was reflected in the way they drew themselves. Marianne drew a profile of a thickset woman, which looked nothing at all like her real, painfully thin self.

The mystery of her weight loss had finally been solved. It would have been tempting for the medical team to have pressed on with increasingly esoteric investigations to explain it, but the answer lay elsewhere. The understanding that psychiatry can bring to a case that seems like a purely physical condition can completely change how a case is managed. Yet sometimes, amid all the technical excellence, scans, scopes, blood tests, and other investigations, the bigger picture can be forgotten. It reminds me of the surgeon's lament that "the operation was a great success, although regrettably the patient died."

Of all the illnesses I see regularly, anorexia nervosa is one of the most puzzling. People have starved themselves for centuries, although in early descriptions they seem to have done it because of religious conviction rather than for the reasons that we now associate with anorexia. Academic textbooks and papers suggest hundreds of theories to account for the illness. A fear of fatness is a central theme, and anorexia is undoubtedly more common in professions where being overweight would be a disadvantage, such as among models and ballet dancers. Genetic studies have examined differences in the rates of anorexia between identical and nonidentical twins. Since identical twins share exactly the same genes as well as the same home environment, and nonidentical twins share the same home environment but have different genes, any differences between the rates of anorexia in identical and nonidentical twin pairs are likely to be accounted for by genetics. And there does appear to be an inherited component to anorexia, because identical twins are more likely to develop it than nonidentical twins. We also know that rigid, obsessional, or perfectionist people are more likely to develop the illness. Other studies have concluded that anorexia is a means by which individuals try to control their family by directing all their family's focus onto their illness.

Yet underlying all this is the core belief among anorexic women that reflects a wider social view—the idea that thinness is a great virtue. This is a peculiarly Western belief not shared by other cultures. For all the work on genetics, types of personality and upbringing, and other relevant factors, without this strange belief that being thin indicates beauty, vigor, sexual attractiveness, and success, there would be no such illness as anorexia nervosa.

As a society, we have a long-held belief in the "ideal shape" or the "perfect body." In times gone by, when the general population barely had enough to eat, being overweight was associated with wealth and prosperity. Now, with industrialized food production and the availability of cheap, high-calorie fast food, wealth and success are instead indicated by being slim and immaculate. The arrival of "size 0" models in the early 2000s caused a crisis, because it showcased a lifestyle that young women admired and wanted to emulate, and deaths from anorexia followed. It got so bad that a number of countries, including France, Italy, Israel, and Spain passed legislation that prohibited models with an unhealthy body mass index from taking part in fashion shows. Even aside from fashion, the portrayal of women in the media favors a particular body shape, and because of Western cultural dominance, we seem to be exporting anorexia to other countries and cultures through television, movies, magazines, and social media.

One of the most unusual studies I read on the subject, published in *The British Journal of Psychiatry*, was carried out on the South Pacific island of Fiji. It was the sort of study that could not easily be repeated, because of a specific set of circumstances in Fiji at that time: there was no widespread use of television. The authors examined the attitudes of adolescent girls concerning their weight and body shape before television was introduced in the 1990s, and then again afterward. They found that exposure to television led to an increase in disordered eating, as a means of losing weight to model themselves on television characters. These were girls who had been content with life before the introduction of television, yet who suddenly became dissatisfied with their body shape. I found the results of this study both predictable and dispiriting, and it helps to explain why the rate of eating disorders in the West has increased with exposure to television, the internet, and social media.

Research into anorexia is carried out for reasons more compelling than simple medical curiosity. People are often surprised to find out that along with substance abuse, anorexia has the highest mortality rate of any mental illness. A sufferer is at least five to ten times more likely to die than someone of their age and gender who is not anorexic. If the illness does not lead to death, starvation affects every single organ system in the body and can lead to anemias, brittle bones, kidney impairment, muscle pain and weakness, stomach problems, difficulty regulating temperature, heart problems, mineral deficiencies in the blood, dry skin, and the collection of fluid in the body, among other problems.

The treatment of anorexia, as in Marianne's case, can be difficult, and the illness can rumble on for many years, with patients often relapsing. When I was a medical student, anorexics were treated on general psychiatry wards alongside patients who had mental illnesses very different from theirs. At that time, a form of a reward system was often used to encourage weight gain: gain one kilogram and you could earn a pair of slippers to wear on the ward, two kilograms and it was a morning paper, three kilograms and you could wear your own clothes, and so forth. This approach has now been stopped, because there is some evidence that patients with anorexia are not sensitive to reward systems, and that weight gains made during a hospital stay are not sustained when patients are discharged. However, the biggest problem with this approach is that it came to be seen as punitive and dehumanizing, with patients being deprived of "privileges" that any person in a hospital might reasonably expect.

This sort of treatment has been replaced by specialist anorexia wards that emphasize normalizing eating in a social context, through education and psychological approaches, with staff and patients sitting down to eat together. In Marianne's case, there was tension between the medical and psychiatric ward regarding who was best placed to manage her care. As often happens in cases where medical and psychiatric issues overlap, the medical team felt they lacked the skills to manage a patient who was "psychiatric," and the psychiatry team felt unequipped to admit a patient who had a need for more complex medical care and refeeding. Marianne was eventually discharged to the care of the local anorexia team, where she was offered individual therapy, as well as support from a specialist nurse. Meals were taken with others seated at the table to normalize eating. This approach helped her gain weight steadily, and when I later bumped into her eating disorders consultant and asked after her, I learned that she had managed to maintain the weight.

Unless it is extreme or causing ill health, anorexia is commonly overlooked. Those people with an eating disorder often do not ask for help, since they do not see it as a problem. Indeed, the condition is sometimes incidental to the patient's referral. My experience with Marianne and many other patients like her has caused me to reflect on the ways in which women are held to particular standards of beauty that lead to much unhappiness and ill health. There is a shame associated with not looking like the aspirational ideal, which leads people to various medical clinics, and less often directly to a psychiatrist, as people usually assume that their problems are physical rather than psychological. Then, of course, there are the efforts to enhance looks through injections, fillers, dyes, and other procedures. Whether women's looks are actually enhanced by all of this is a question of perspective, but it takes a brave teenage girl to reject the powerful social norms.

Over time, men have also been drawn into a similar pattern of behavior. A few years ago, at the end of a busy afternoon clinic, I saw a young man called Theo, who was in his late twenties and had been referred to me by his dermatologist. On the way to my office from the waiting room, he seemed uncomfortable and distracted. He entered my room uneasily, as if this was the last place he wanted to be. He was wearing jeans with tears on both knees, a long-sleeved T-shirt, and a baseball cap. He was of average height and had a somewhat diffident manner; if you'd seen him on the street, I doubt you would have guessed that he was suffering as he was. His problem was new to me; he had an overwhelming, all-encompassing, and near-paralyzing fear of going bald.

I glanced at the letter from the dermatologist who had referred Theo to me. He had tried to reassure Theo that he was worrying for nothing, telling him that he was showing no signs of male-pattern baldness. Nevertheless, Theo's anxiety had persisted, and it must have been infectious, because the dermatologist, despite stating that treatment was not necessary, had prescribed medication to encourage hair growth.

My encounter with Theo drew me into the parallel universe in which he was living. He believed that he was destined to live a life of loneliness and rejection, a fate to which he was unable to reconcile himself. He thought about his hair constantly, searching online for hair-loss remedies several times every day. This activity brought him only transient relief, yet he was unable to stop himself from doing it.

Furthermore, the world seemed to be conspiring against Theo to reinforce his anxieties. He had seen an advertisement about male-pattern baldness on the London Underground that was difficult to avoid: an aerial view of a man's thinning hairline, and pictures of the same satisfied man taken later to demonstrate "success." I had myself heard something on the radio that same week, along the lines of "Do you suffer from male-pattern baldness?" The implication was that you couldn't simply be bald without "suffering" from it, as if baldness was a newly discovered disease.

I started to go bald in my twenties, and by the time I was married in my mid-thirties, my baldness was quite advanced. I remember where I was when I noticed it for the first time. It was in a clothes store in Camden Town. Near the till, the shop had a black-and-white CCTV image, visible on a monitor. It would fade to white every few seconds, before displaying an image from a different store camera. I found myself strangely entranced by the screen and tried to work out, as the picture gradually developed definition, where in the shop it was. After the third or fourth change of view, I remember seeing the screen turn from white to show another view of the shop from high up, with a few people scattered about, one motionless. As the picture sharpened, the top of the head of the motionless customer showed a lighter patch on the crown, and simultaneously I realized that it was me. Yet it had never occurred to me to mind going bald—it was just something that happened. While I was discussing whether baldness was going to ruin Theo's life, I wondered if he saw the irony of having this conversation with a bald doctor. I thought about a joke Larry David once told: "Anyone can be confident with a full head of hair. But a confident bald man—there's your diamond in the rough."

The hair industry is the only winner in this situation, having perpetuated the idea that men should have a full head of hair, as a sign of confidence, attractiveness, and masculinity. And men have started to buy into it, creating a global industry that trades on their insecurity. One can easily imagine the fear of baldness being added to the next incarnation of the psychiatric classification system, thereby legitimizing an invented illness and encouraging hapless balding men to pay for their hair treatment along with their psychiatric care.

We seem to be creating an equivalent of anorexia nervosa in men, relating to an arbitrary view of perfection in hair. However, perhaps it is not quite as arbitrary as it first appears; what both hair and thinness have in common is that they are the properties of youth. When I was growing up, there was no market in men's beauty products nor even in men's fashion. Men used shaving products, but it took an ex-heavyweight boxer, Henry Cooper, to persuade them in an advertising campaign that they would not be emasculated by wearing Brut aftershave. Today the men's beauty market, often referred to as "male grooming," is predicted to be worth globally around $81 billion by 2024. While concern about appearance is nothing new, and men have previously worried to the point of preoccupation about such things as penis size or body build, these new social pressures have extended the range of concerns that men now have into areas that were previously considered feminine. This has increased the range of insecurities that men have started to develop. The number of male patients who come to my clinic with concerns about their appearance is a trickle rather than a flood, yet it feels like a change that will work its way through society, to the benefit of nobody except the industries that make money out of these insecurities.

Theo's anxiety about baldness would fall under what is generally termed body dysmorphic disorder. First described as "dysmorphophobia" by the Italian physician Enrico Morselli in the late nineteenth century, it is a psychiatric problem in which sufferers possess a sustained focus on a particular part of the body, accompanied by an implacable belief that this perceived imperfection makes them defective or unattractive. The individual's worries about this unwanted aspect of their appearance quickly become all-consuming and can end up dominating their life. In Theo's case, this included his carrying a mirror with him at all times to check for any change or progression in his hairline during the day. Even during my consultation with him, Theo came to my side of the desk, bent his head toward me, and asked whether in my opinion he was going bald—even though he had only recently been reassured by a dermatologist.

Theo's treatment was time-consuming and not entirely successful, which is not unusual in conditions like this, particularly where it is severe or has gone on for a long time before the patient sought help. Sometimes the best that can be hoped for is that the preoccupation becomes more manageable, although inevitably it worsens at times of stress. I prescribed medication for his anxiety and obsessional behaviors, but he was ambivalent about taking it and soon stopped. The other part of his treatment was cognitive behavioral therapy, which in his case included working through the many falsehoods going unchallenged in his own mind, such as the belief that no woman could ever find a bald man attractive. He clung to this notion despite overwhelming evidence to the contrary, as even a quick perusal of the celebrity gossip columns would have demonstrated. It took much time and patience to persuade him of this, and though he eventually accepted it at an intellectual level, he did not seem to believe it emotionally.

We also worked on response prevention, with the aim of preventing him from repeatedly checking his hairline and asking those close to him for reassurance. The hope was that it would lessen his anxiety, since anxiety of this sort will often intensify and then abate naturally, without the need for reassurance. This can then lead to a sense of control over the situation that has hitherto been lacking. I also suggested that he try to engage normally with the world, rather than hiding himself away. He would soon discover that nobody minded about his baldness apart from him. He would, I hoped, gradually habituate to a new normal in which the many distractions of daily life would shift his focus away from his hair. Throughout his treatment he was set back by all sorts of reminders (one week, he showed me a newspaper feature that asked whether we will ever see "a cure for baldness," which reinforced his view that baldness was an unwelcome disease that might be cured).

I think of the many ways in which health anxieties find their way into my clinics, most commonly via other specialists, and about how much of a doctor's work is to define where "normal" stops and where illness begins. The borders are far more porous and blurred than is commonly believed, which is why judgment is such a valuable skill in doctors, who need to define where social anxieties end and medicine begins. The trickiest thing, and the biggest challenge to the medical system, is that this boundary is constantly changing, influenced by societal changes and expectations. Symptoms can quickly go from being an observed phenomenon to a recognized condition with an effective treatment. This has happened recently with gender dysphoria. People who felt that they had been born into the wrong gender were in the past ignored, then seen as exhibiting a perversion. Now there is an increasing acceptance of the diverse ways in which gender is experienced, and hormonal treatments and gender reassignment surgery have become accepted. Similarly, homosexuality was defined as an illness right up until 1973, before disappearing from the American diagnostic manual in 1987. Prior to that, it was considered to be a treatable psychiatric condition, and gay men would be shown pictures of naked men while a small electric shock was administered to the thumb, in an attempt to break the link between seeing naked men and pleasure. Medicine, psychiatry, and social change are constantly rubbing up against one another, and I often find myself at the center of this.

In my clinical practice, while there are many different ways in which doctors and therapists relate to patients, I often reflect on the work of Carl Rogers, an important, although now largely forgotten, figure of twentieth-century psychology. Born just outside Chicago in 1902, he studied religion before turning his attentions to the interactions between therapists and their patients. One of his most significant contributions was what he referred to as client-centered therapy. The central idea of this therapy was that we tend to value other people according to our judgment of whether they deserve our respect. If people do not achieve according to our societal norms and values—for example, if they don't work or they use drugs—our estimation of them falls, and we no longer respect or value them. Inevitably they then come to see themselves as undeserving of respect and love.

Carl Rogers argued that individuals need love and respect because they are human beings rather than because of what they have achieved or whether we have judged them to be worthy. He called this unconditional positive regard and maintained that in any interaction, the doctor or therapist needed to be genuine and accepting of the patient for who he or she is. Of all the schools of therapy that I have affinity for, Carl Rogers's speaks to me most. We all have a fundamental need to feel respected and valued, to feel that we matter—not because of our appearance, the job we have, or the clothes we wear, but because we are human beings.

This is why I find patients such as Marianne and Theo so emotionally challenging. We have created a society where superficial things like appearance, cars, hair, and money have become the standard by which people judge themselves and others. The result is evident in my clinics: anxious, unhappy people who feel worthless and project their anxieties onto their appearance. They often end up in various medical clinics trying to correct their "deficit." Baldness carries no intrinsic meaning except as a normal sign of maleness. The fact that we have imbued baldness with such a negative meaning tells us something about our view of aging and perhaps about the place of the elderly in our society. Whether patients are seeing plastic surgeons, dermatologists, or psychiatrists about these superficial concerns, their presentation to health services at all represents a fundamental flaw in our society.

PAIN

It struck me at medical school how life is experienced by humans. Every thought, every experience, all our ambitions, every sensation, from the smell of a rose to the awe of seeing the Grand Canyon, from the first flush of romance to the frustration of a canceled flight—all these sensations and emotions are experienced simply as electrical impulses across cell membranes. Billions of crackling nerve fibers release chemical transmitters into the tiny spaces between nerves, to promote or inhibit the firing of the next one, in an orchestra so exquisite and complex that it is likely to remain forever beyond human comprehension. I feel awe at the endless complexity of the human brain, and despair at our ever understanding its workings and its secrets. Are we, in all our hopes, fears, aspirations and ambitions, just a network of neurons? Would it be possible, if we had enough computer power, to build an exact replica of the human brain? Or is the "brain as computer" just a twenty-first-century conceptualization? My closest friend Alex Leff, a professor of neurology, once told me that he thought of the brain as a mirror, simply reflecting back to us what we thought it did, and that our research just tends to confirm what we were looking for in the first place.

Brain function has been the subject of various theories over time. Aristotle, the ancient Greek philosopher, maintained that the brain acted as a cooling system for heat produced by the heart, with its vast network of blood vessels acting like a radiator. Over the ages the brain was seen as the seat of the soul or as a complicated control center for the physical working of the body. As time passed, the consensus developed that the brain was divided into specific areas of function.

The person initially most closely associated with this theory was Franz Gall, an eighteenth-century physician. Although there was (and is) some truth in the localization of brain areas, Gall's theory was wrong in two significant respects. The first error was in his being too specific in what the brain areas did—for example, believing that there were brain areas for things like kindness or greed or caution. The second error was in believing that the skull expanded to reflect the underlying brain area, so someone with a high work ethic, for example, would have a prominence of their skull in that area, and someone with foresight a prominence over that part of the brain, and so forth. This led to the pseudoscience of phrenology, in which physicians claimed to know someone's character from the shape of their skull.

Phrenology became very popular in Europe and the United States, and it's not hard to see its appeal, because it provides a coherent and easily measurable assessment of personality. At least one reason I have heard for why psychiatrists are sometimes called shrinks is that their therapy would contract the swollen area of brain with the undesirable characteristic, and the overlying bit of skull would similarly shrink down over it. But as is true of most medical theories throughout history, which enjoy their brief period of popularity followed by being discredited and cast aside, by the nineteenth century, phrenology was obsolete, and the mysteries of the brain once again remained an unanswered question.

In the modern era, the brain is conceptualized as a highly intricate computer with vast systems of integrated networks, although with broad localization of some brain functions such as movement, sensation, and language. Yet no computer model could explain consciousness or higher levels of brain function like abstract thought. This has led some to postulate a quantum theory of brain function to better explain the unexplainable. It is an interesting theory and difficult to prove (or disprove), although I suspect that two things you don't really understand, such as quantum mechanics and brain function, will usually look the same to you.

When it comes to understanding how pain is experienced, there has been some progress. Yet the ways most doctors conceptualize and treat pain are stuck in a bygone era. The vertiginous anatomy lecture theater, just off the quaintly named Tennis Court Road in Cambridge, was also reminiscent of a bygone era. This was where I attended anatomy and physiology lectures several times a week during my undergraduate years. The anatomy lecture theater was wooden paneled and steep. With its musty smell etched deep into the fabric of the building, it seemed to contain the ghosts of past generations of doctors. In that very lecture theater, we had a lecture that I suspect had been given to many generations of medical students.

We were told that pain was a symptom of tissue damage. Descartes, a seventeenth-century French philosopher, had proposed this model. The pain then traveled through nerves, which Descartes imagined as hollow tubes carrying "animal spirits" up to the brain. This is in broad essence what I was being taught some three hundred years later. When a part of the body is damaged or injured, chemicals are released from nerve endings, which stimulates the nerve fibers, and from there messages pass upward to the brain. Interestingly, that lecture was the first time I had heard that pain passes along two different types of nerve fibers on its way to the brain. The first type is A nerve fibers, fast fibers that quickly relay to the brain the sensation of something painful. Pain is also carried along the slower C fibers, which carry deeper and more specific pain information. These two different types of fibers account for why, when you put your hands under a scalding-hot tap, there is an "Ah!" as you realize the tap is too hot and you withdraw your hand (the A fibers), followed by a longer and more pained "Owww" as the pain reaches the brain a fraction of a second later via the C fibers, causing a deeper and more profound sense of pain.

In an often-cited paper from the 1960s, pain researchers Ronald Melzack and Patrick Wall proposed that there operates some sort of gate mechanism in the spinal cord, an access point that either allows pain signals to travel up the brain to the spinal cord (when the gate is open) or closes the gate off to pain. When pain is experienced in a part of the body—for example, when you get hit on the arm—information travels along nerve pathways to the spinal cord, and at the spinal cord there is a kind of junction that determines whether pain signals will pass upward into the brain. One of the elements in the decision as to whether pain will travel up the spinal cord and on into the brain is touch. A light touch to the painful area (in our example, the arm) sends the touch sensation along nerve pathways, and this light touch blocks the pain fiber signal at the spinal cord "gate." This theory makes intuitive sense, when you consider that our first reaction when we bang our shin against a low table is to rub it, using the light touch to inhibit the pain fibers from accessing the spinal cord. It also explains why "kissing it better," providing a light touch when a child injures himself, prevents pain transmission, and may not be simply an old wives' tale.

So acute pain is, in some respects at least, easy to understand. This is because pain follows well-delineated pathways from the injured organ, traveling along nerve fibers to eventually reach the spinal cord. The spinal cord then serves as the main motorway for transmission of signals through the body, and like the M1 motorway in the UK, the spinal cord goes from north to south. The nerves that run down the spinal cord carry messages down from the brain, and outward at each level of the spinal cord, into the body. The opposite also takes place. Messages and sensations from the body pass into the spinal cord at the segment for that part of the body and then up into the brain. At the brain the electrical signals from the nerves are decoded, and we experience the nerve signals as a sensation—in this case, as pain.

The sudden pain involved in getting your toe trodden on or in smashing into a glass door that you didn't realize was there is an example of what is known as acute pain. This is to distinguish it from chronic pain. People are often confused about the meaning of the term "chronic pain"; many patients that I see understand this to mean extreme pain, whereas what "chronic" actually refers to here is pain that has gone on for some time, by convention lasting for longer than three months (named after Chronos, the personification of time in ancient Greek mythology).

For a psychiatrist, though, explaining the terminology isn't the problem. The biggest source of error is the widespread belief that chronic pain is exactly the same as acute pain, only it has lasted longer. This misunderstanding is just as common among doctors as among their patients, and the treatment failures that result from this misunderstanding are a significant source of referrals to my clinic.

But if chronic pain is not the same as acute pain, then what is it? Irene Tracey is a researcher at Oxford who has been looking into chronic pain. Along with her colleague Catherine Bushnell, she proposes that chronic pain can be thought of as its own separate disease, with particular changes in brain structure and function in those people who suffer with chronic pain. Chronic pain does not always have to have a physical cause somewhere in the body. Phantom limb pain, where an individual feels pain in a limb that has been amputated, is a strange but well-recognized phenomenon.

Patients with persistent pain do eventually end up in my clinic, though. I met Majid for the first time in an unusually quiet clinic one July afternoon. The waiting room was absolutely sweltering. The secretary was caught between keeping the single fan in her unbearably hot office or moving it into the waiting room, which is what she eventually did. Even with the fan, though, the sun was beating in through the floor-to-ceiling glass front of our psychiatry offices. People stared listlessly at posters on the wall advising them about how to complain or outlining how to identify the symptoms of bird flu. I had by then, that far into summer, abandoned my usual suit and tie, and was in a short-sleeved shirt and chinos, the standard doctor's summer wardrobe, finished off with socks and brogues. I still felt weighed down and stickily hot, and envied the female doctors, who were wearing light summer dresses and sandals.

Sitting in a chair, wiping sweat off his forehead with a handkerchief loosely bunched in his tremulous hand, sat Majid. A cloud of aftershave hung over him, so strong that it was almost visible, like smog over Beijing. He was wearing loose-fitting trousers and an open-neck short-sleeved shirt and sandals with socks. His hair was sparse, oiled and pulled into a part on the side that began just above one ear. Scrupulously correct and charming, he looked to be in his thirties, and when he spoke, his heavily accented words seemed to glide together in smooth, toneless waves. His moustache quivered as he spoke. He walked effortfully to the clinic room while I engaged him in small talk about the hot weather. His hand flapped as he guided himself along the banister of the narrow corridor and then into my office, where he sat down at the chair next to the desk, grimacing with pain.

After the pleasantries were complete, we began the interview by talking about his background. He told me that he had been born in Kabul to a fairly middle-class family. His father had a position in a government hospital, and his mother stayed at home to look after him and his four siblings. He had spent his childhood in Afghanistan. He lamented that his country had never been free of outside interference, although he recalled his upbringing in Kabul as a happy time in his life. He himself went abroad to university and trained as a civil engineer, before returning to work on various construction projects to help rebuild his shattered country.

During a working trip somewhere in the wide expanse of the country, his party was ambushed and kidnapped. He remembered that one of the group was seriously injured in the initial assault, but he didn't find out until much later that his colleague had died. In the meantime, he was taken and held hostage in a tiny room somewhere in the parched Afghan wilderness. He recalled the humiliation of being stripped naked and the pain of being beaten, accompanied by the fear and helplessness he felt in his predicament. He was moved around frequently over the following weeks and resigned himself to his fate, weary of the fear that he felt but never quite free of it. The days dragged by, and he noticed the pain increasing in his chest, where he had been repeatedly hit during the initial kidnapping, and the pain in his leg where he had been chained.

He told me that eventually a ransom was paid and he was released by his kidnappers. He had lost seven kilograms (fifteen pounds) in weight, and recalls feeling bewildered, scared, and humiliated. After a lengthy journey, he reached the relative safety of Kabul. He found it hard to settle there, lost interest in his work, and together with his family decided it would be preferable if he made a new start in the UK.

He told me how beautiful his country was, and how gray and unwelcoming Britain seemed to him. He said wistfully that he missed Afghanistan. Life in the UK had been difficult. He'd had to seek asylum, and he had a hard time finding work. He felt a sense of failure in his inability to provide for his family and ended up driving shifts in a minicab. His house was damp in the winter, and currently he had a problem controlling ants in the kitchen. His pain, particularly his chest pain, was becoming a constant bother, and he sought help from his doctor. His GP, initially concerned that the pain might be from his heart, had done some tests, sending him for chest X- rays and ECGs. The results came back negative, yet the pain intensified and began to radiate down one arm, which became affected by tremors. His leg continued to ache. Running out of possibilities and with no clear diagnosis to treat, his doctor prescribed painkillers, although these had no effect. With some hesitation on the part of the GP, stronger painkillers were used, which helped initially, but then the effect seemed to wear off, and Majid was back to square one, only now addicted to opiate medication.

Over the following months, he was seen in cardiology with a diagnosis of "atypical chest pain," but after several appointments over a period of months, they lost interest and discharged him, with "no cardiac cause." He was seen in rheumatology and then neurology, each time with blood and other types of tests that did not show any cause for his pain. Finally, he was referred to the pain clinic, who tried valiantly with different medications and combinations of treatments, but to no avail. Majid accepted all of his treatments with courtesy, but without enthusiasm or expectation, and now eighteen months later, seemingly for want of something better to try, he was referred to me.

Persistent pain is always an interesting referral for a general hospital psychiatrist. It has a number of contributing factors that do not relate to the usual things one thinks about when considering pain. Research done in the 1950s and 1960s demonstrated that one's culture is linked with how pain was experienced. In a famous experiment in the United States in the 1950s, Mark Zborowski selected ethnocultural groups of volunteers in New York. The main focus of the study was on volunteers who were either Jewish, Italian, or "Old Americans" (typically white Protestants). All of them currently had a painful condition, the majority experiencing back pain from slipped disks or other spinal problems. The groups were selected because Italians and Jews were thought to exaggerate pain, and the "Old Americans" acted as a kind of control group, against which the other cultures could be compared.

The researchers found that while Italian Americans and Jewish patients both had an emotional response to pain, Italian Americans were concerned primarily about the experience of pain itself, whereas Jewish patients focused more on what the pain meant for their health and their future. This was reflected in their attitudes toward pain relief, so that Italian Americans were more accepting of painkillers, whilst the Jewish patients were concerned about dependency, and moreover whether the medication would simply mask an underlying disease process that was being left untreated. This meant that when Jewish patients were relieved of pain, their worries did not resolve, and their trust in doctors was not necessarily enhanced. The researchers found that "Old Americans" liked to talk about their pain unemotionally, offering a descriptive and factual account of the pain ("the detached role of an unemotional observer") to help the doctors perform their function optimally in diagnosing it. These patients believed that being emotional about pain only hindered that process. So it seems that for the same painful condition, there is a cultural difference in how the pain is experienced and communicated.

But what of pain threshold, the point at which pain is experienced? In a 1960s study, electric shocks were administered to volunteers to explore pain thresholds. American Protestants, Irish Americans, and Jewish groups were tested and found to be similar in their pain tolerance. Since the Jewish volunteers knew the cause of the pain, they were not so concerned by the why of the pain itself, which helped them tolerate the pain much better. We have probably all had a similar experience, in which knowing that the cause of pain is not serious makes it hurt far less. Spontaneous chest pain is much more anxiety producing, and therefore much more painful, than pain caused by a tennis ball's striking our chest. This tells us something about the meaning of pain and its influence on our perception of pain. A similar study about the same time showed that Jewish subjects were shown to have a lower pain threshold—that is, until they were told that the experiment was to see which religious group could tolerate the greatest pain. The knowledge increased their pain threshold substantially. All of this goes to demonstrate that when we experience a painful stimulus, the meaning of the pain and our emotions play a far greater role than we like to think in how the pain is actually experienced.

The description of pain varies from culture to culture, as summarized in "Ethnocultural Variations in Pain," a fascinating chapter included in a book about pain. In one study mentioned in this chapter, Irish volunteers tended to avoid pain language, so instead of saying how much, say, their eye hurt, they would use an expression like "the pain is like sand in my eye." Italian subjects, on the other hand, reported more widespread symptoms in more bodily locations and found the pains more disabling. Japanese patients are said to express pain in concise and relatively restricted language, such as describing the pain as either intense or not intense; shallow or deep; horizontally extended or confined. The English language often uses metaphor to describe pain (and this is certainly my experience of talking to patients in clinic): pain is described as "burning," "shooting," or "stabbing," for example. And any consideration of the ways people describe their pain leads to the inevitable question: Does the way you describe your pain, including the language you use to speak about it, influence the way you experience it? I believe that a lot of these cultural differences from experiments done in the 1960s have been watered down over the years as cultures have assimilated, and undoubtedly the differences between cultures are not quite as clear-cut in real life as in experimental designs. But what is clear is that there is little objective measure of pain, and some of the many contributory factors in how we experience pain are the culture we come from, the language we speak, and the meaning that the pain has for us.

There are other factors, too. One of them relates to our assessment of pain and what it means, often referred to as Bayesian probability. This describes our own subjective estimates of probabilities and risk that may cause us to revise our thinking in light of new information. This is different from normal probability, which look at situations in which the odds are known, as when we know that the chances of heads in a coin flip are one in two.

But what if the probabilities are not entirely known? What if the question is, *How likely is this pain in my hand to have a serious cause?* You may already have a few pieces of information. You may have had a number of investigations that are all normal, which of course is encouraging. But you may also have a belief that if there is pain somewhere in your body, then there must be a cause, even if the doctors cannot find it. So let's say you start with a figure in your mind of 75 percent probability that the pain is serious, and given that likelihood, moving or exercising your hand is going to cause damage.

You also have other information, such as the feedback from the pain receptors in your hand, that can modify your belief in there being a serious cause. If the pain is fairly mild, it may reduce your estimate of the probability of a serious cause, so that you decide not to worry about it. And if the pain is intense when you move your hand, you may modify the probability of a serious cause upward—say, to 90 percent.

What happens, though, if your prior expectation about there being a serious cause of hand pain is wrong? What if the real answer is close to 1 percent that there is a serious cause, and not the 75 percent you initially believed? Do you correct your belief based on feedback from your hand ("it's not so painful; perhaps I was worried about nothing") and revise your probability of a serious cause downward? Or do you distort the feedback from your hand because you so strongly believe in a serious cause ("I mustn't move my hand at all; any movement is bound to be really painful")? In other words, are we more likely to believe the evidence from our senses, or are we more likely to believe what we think is true? My experience suggests it is the latter. The higher your "top-down" prediction from your brain, the more you will distort the reality of the pain receptors from your hand, so that any movement of the hand will cause pain. In other words, our brain prefers what it thinks to be true and distorts reality to fit that expectation.

Eventually, we need to make a firm and final decision about how serious the cause of the hand pain is. If the belief is strong in the beginning, then the final decision the brain makes is that there is a serious cause. All sensations from that area will now be distorted to feel more painful, and the hand gets used less and less, further amplifying the pain when it eventually gets used, which serves only to reconfirm the hypothesis that there is something seriously wrong.

In fact, if you have ever wondered why placebos work, it is exactly because of this scenario, only in reverse. A placebo is a medication with no active ingredients, although it can have powerful effects, and interestingly many individuals given placebos even report side effects. Certainly placebos can be helpful in treating pain of this sort. When patients are given a placebo, the top-down belief that they develop is that their pain will start to improve. This means that the bottom-up sensations from the nerves in the hand (in our case) are interpreted as being less painful. This leads to the hand's being used more, and the brain becomes more and more aware that the sensations are not in fact painful, which reinforces the belief that the pain is resolving, probably not serious, and getting better. The top-down decision from the brain soon becomes "the pain is resolving, the tablet is working," and in time, little attention is paid to the previously painful hand, which now starts to work normally.

This can be difficult to explain in a busy clinic, because it goes back to why people have the beliefs that they do. We do not start off each day with an unbiased view of the world or our bodies. We wake up each day with a preconceived set of expectations about the world, beliefs rarely changed by the evidence around us. As an example, someone paranoid by nature will believe people are paying them more attention when they are out on the street or will think they are being jostled more in a crowd, even when objectively this isn't true.

I have seen this firsthand, having had the rather unsettling experience of walking through a virtual reality library, used as the setting to demonstrate exactly this point. As I moved through the virtual library, avatars sitting at the desks would look up, in a fairly neutral way, as I walked by the tables that they were working at. When some individuals in a trial were asked to walk through exactly the same virtual reality library, with the same figures looking up at them, they saw these benign figures, the very ones I had seen, as more hostile and threatening. These individuals interpreted the avatars' neutral facial expressions in a mistrustful way. This was further evidence that our beliefs about the world around us distort the reality of what is happening, so that seeing is not believing, and two people can be in exactly the same scenario and assess what has happened in entirely different ways. And where people have preexisting anxiety-inducing beliefs about their body—for example, that all sensations must be taken seriously; that pain must always be a sign of serious disease; that doctors commonly miss serious diagnoses— then all these will reinforce a high state of alert, and pain will flourish.

The other factor that influences pain is mood. Depressed patients experience more physical symptoms, including pain, than nondepressed patients. In fact, in depression, physical symptoms are the norm rather than the exception. And when depressed patients lack motivation, drive, or enthusiasm for life, then they will typically ruminate on the pain itself, with the inevitable result that the pain gets worse. When people are feeling down, dejected, or demoralized, pain is experienced as far more troublesome and more intractable. The effect works in both directions. The experience of ongoing pain becomes even more demoralizing and leads to worsening depression, which then exacerbates the experience of pain, and the negative cycle of depression and pain continues.

Anxiety disorders similarly will feed into this pain cycle. Most patients I see will initially worry about what the pain means, and nowadays they nearly always end up googling the symptoms. I have never, in a career lasting almost thirty years, had a patient search for a symptom and then been reassured that there is nothing to worry about. I am prepared to accept that I see a skewed population of people, and that people who are reassured by their internet search wouldn't end up at their doctor. Yet it seems to be a universal experience: googling a set of symptoms creates more problems than it resolves. For a start, the rarest or most unlikely cause of the symptoms is nearly always what catches the patient's eye, and the anxiety about the cause of the symptoms is reinforced: "My doctor never mentioned that! Perhaps I need a second opinion." This is reminiscent of Samuel Shem's classic novel about junior doctors, in which he comments that when a doctor hears hoofbeats outside the window, he thinks *horse,* but when a medical student hears them, he thinks *zebra.* Google searches for patients with limited medical knowledge largely yield zebra diagnoses. Yet the persistent worry and catastrophic thinking reinforces the top-down belief that something must be wrong and can skew the symptoms that the individual experiences.

There is also evidence that adverse childhood events predispose some patients to developing unexplained pain. One of the biggest studies that looked at this was the 1958 cohort. The 1958 cohort is a population of over 17,000 people born in a single week in 1958. They have been followed up closely over many years, for all sorts of problems and conditions. Because so much data has been collected on them over the years, when conditions develop over time, it allows the researchers to look back and see if the individuals who developed the condition had any factors in common. When researchers looked at chronic widespread pain, they found that children who had been in institutional care had an increased risk of developing such pain. This was also true of children who experienced maternal death or financial hardship in childhood. So it seems, in some individuals at least, that the experience of difficulties in childhood makes a difference in how they will develop or experience pain later in life. In fact, adverse childhood experiences are a marker for a range of poor health outcomes, not just for unexplained pain. One large U.S. study showed a relationship between adverse childhood experiences and the development of heart disease, liver disease, cancer, and lung disease. The authors of the study thought it was likely that adverse childhood experiences led to unhealthy coping mechanisms— those that may provide immediate short-term relief while causing long-term damage, such as smoking, alcohol, drug abuse, or multiple sexual partners. These may all provide transient relief from stress and unhappiness, but if they are used as the main source of coping, they lead to persistent ill health and a shortened lifespan.

There were a number of reasons why Majid's painkillers were not working and his pain was resistant to all attempts at treatment. He was clearly very anxious. In fact he had a number of features typical of an anxiety disorder, with anxious ruminations, catastrophic thinking, and a constant sense of foreboding, but he was very resistant to any psychological treatment. He believed that the pain was a consequence of permanent body damage, caused by the abusive treatment handed out by his kidnappers, which the doctors lacked the sophistication (and, he implied, the interest) to find. He was bewildered and offended by the referral to a psychiatrist, although he felt he ought to attend "to prove I'm not mad, Doctor" and thereby be reinstated in the medical clinics that had discharged him, and on to more effective treatments.

As the interview progressed, though, the atmosphere became less tense. After he had talked about the great shame of his kidnap, his fear, his feelings of being unmanned; after he had tried but failed not to cry, hastily wiping his eyes with the back of his hand, he began to feel unburdened, and it became hard to stop him from talking. He talked of his shame at not working and not providing for his family. He talked about his nightmares, in which he dreamed of being kidnapped and tied down, so that he became fearful of going to sleep. He spoke of his heightened state of fear when out on the street, even though he knew nobody was looking for him. He talked of his loneliness away from his country and friends, his inability to connect with others in the UK, and the cultural differences that he had never really gotten over. He went on to discuss the shame of having to come to a psychiatry department like mine, something he never in his life expected to do. And finally, after he had talked well beyond his appointment time, to my great surprise, he asked what I thought about his pain and whether I thought it was psychological.

We met several times over the next few months. Majid always arrived early for his appointments, approaching them with an intellectualized voice of inquiry, still skeptical of a psychological formulation of his pain. He most of all enjoyed discussing Bayesian probability, which he felt was an intellectual and abstract enough concept of pain to be unthreatening, and which he was able to concede might have some merit. We tried distraction techniques, to help him focus his attention away from his pain, to see whether this would override his anxieties about what the pain was and temporarily suspend his top-down beliefs that his pain was serious and progressive. We also talked about probability, and whether the fact that the doctors had failed to find a serious cause of his pain meant that there was no serious cause, or whether it was still likely, as he believed, that the doctors had missed something. We rationally examined the evidence both for and against these postulates, evidence he now saw was greatly in favor of no serious cause. We discussed how he could integrate into society and build a life here, and how he could develop a renewed sense of purpose. Throughout all of this, we avoided talking directly about emotions, such as his anxiety disorder, because it made him uncomfortable. Indeed, any discussion of anti-anxiety medication led to a lengthy and intellectualized discussion on neurotransmitters and pain pathways, and my answers never really convinced him anyway.

Over time, he began to cut down on the pain medication, which he said in any case was making him tired, until he stopped taking it altogether "as an experiment," which appealed to his scientific nature. The appointments became less frequent, as eventually Majid declared himself better. He still worried about the pain coming back, about all the what-ifs, but with his wife now pregnant (he'd kept that quiet), he felt that he needed to move on, and he could always contact me in the future if he needed.

I never heard directly from him again, although he did call my secretary to say that he'd had a daughter. But it struck me that despite the cultural differences and the unhappy story that had brought him to see me, his case was quite typical. Once he had overcome the awkwardness of being referred to a psychiatrist, he was gradually able to understand a different conceptualization of his pain that over time began to make sense, so that my suggestions seemed rational. It's fair to say that he was never prepared to accept that he had an anxiety disorder, but psychiatry, like the rest of medicine, is about finding a way, and to my great delight, Majid got there in the end.

WISHING FOR THE END

Unusually for me, my office is tidy. My papers are neatly stacked and my pens are lined up a little obsessively along the grains of fake wood on my cheap but expansive Formica desk, which also houses a large NHS-issue desktop computer. I find that a mess when I am working makes me feel a little agitated and overwhelmed (and by contrast at home, where my priority is to be relaxed and comfortable, I barely notice when things are untidy). So my office has become for me an oasis of calm. It has a coffee machine on a little table, lots of colored coffee pods in a bowl, some chunky mugs that I have grown unreasonably attached to, and a see-through kettle that I failed to anticipate after a single use would become coated in scale.

I breathe easily, having finished my clinic and uploaded my clinic letters to the ether, from which they will return, typed, later the same day. This, I thought, is one of the few instances in my life when technology has made my life easier. Today, at my tidy desk, I prepared to enjoy a treat. It was my regular Monday bonus because I have a clinic in the morning and one in the afternoon, and supervise one of my junior doctors at lunchtime. In my free twenty minutes of the day, like a seal at the zoo, I perform better if there's a treat. And like the seal, my treat today was raw fish, sushi being something I have discovered later in life. I unwrapped the box, pondered what to do with the notional "salad" garnish (is it for eating or decoration?), and was mixing the soy sauce with wasabi when there was a knock at my door. My sushi lay just out of reach on my desk for the remainder of the afternoon, giving my room a fishy smell that I noticed only when I returned later in the day.

It was my registrar, who wanted to discuss an urgent referral. It had come from the oncology team, who deal with all types of cancers in the hospital. The patient, April, was a woman in her early fifties with a lung cancer that would be fatal if left untreated. At this stage it wasn't too late, albeit the treatment involved some unpleasant chemotherapy and radiotherapy. She was currently an inpatient on the oncology ward and had told the oncologists that she had made up her mind that she didn't want to have any further medical care.

I headed over to the ward to see April, uneasy as I always am when thinking about the consequences of a treatment refusal like hers. I felt the burden of knowing that a job well done could lead to a chance of life, and a clumsy or badly handled consultation could have fatal consequences. Once on the ward, I checked that the dayroom was free and invited April there. Hospital dayrooms are intended to provide patients with somewhere else to be aside from their hospital bed. The room is usually sparsely furnished with some armchairs or sofas, and sometimes a few books are stacked on the windowsill. There's rarely anyone in the dayroom, though, and as usual it was empty when I arrived on the ward. I gestured toward the dayroom sofa, where April sat to one side of it, and I sat down facing her, in the too-big armchair.

I started the consultation by keeping away from anything too contentious, asking her to tell me a bit about her background. April was originally from the south coast of England and had what is usually referred to as an alternative lifestyle. She was somewhat scornful of what I represented, which is to say the staid, conventional, repressed, unimaginative, and socially conservative world of the medical profession. It took her some time to get beyond this and engage in the discussion we were having. And in fairness, it took me some time to see past the tie-dyed loose-fitting trousers, bangles, and sandals. I thought of protest camps, and her nose ring made me think of an Aberdeen Angus. I don't believe most doctors have a problem with alternative lifestyles, but rather the difficulty for doctors is in respecting alternative health beliefs, particularly when they lead to the shortening of life. I have always wondered why real medicines are subject to lengthy and expensive trials to measure effectiveness and safety before they can be prescribed, but it is possible to make pretty well any claim you want about alternative remedies and sell them directly to the public without producing any data about safety or effectiveness.

So, with each of us armed with a full set of prejudices, I began to take April's case history. As we got talking, I warmed to her. She was sharp, witty, and self-aware, with a self-deprecating sense of humor. I think the feeling was mutual. We had led completely divergent lives but were bound together by a common humanity, and as it turns out a similar sense of humor, which led to a mutual understanding, liking, and respect. We talked about her unconventional childhood: she was moved regularly from place to place as a girl, and for a time lived in a woman's refuge with her mother to escape her abusive father. She left school, lived in London on a houseboat for a time, and then had moved into various squats and communes. She made her living designing jewelry that she sold at markets on the weekend. We were the same age, and I thought back to my childhood in suburban Manchester. I thought about my prep school, followed by an independent grammar school, followed by university. I thought of the safety and security of my upbringing, and what I had seen then as both conventional and boring now seemed like a blessing. I wondered how I would have turned out if I'd lived April's life. Probably not as well as she had, I expect. She had never wanted to marry or settle down, and had said that she really did not trust men, hastily adding with a laugh that as a doctor I didn't really count as a man. Which led to more laughter when she realized how that sounded. We talked for some time, and then she came to the real reason she wanted to see me. It was not about alternative as opposed to conventional treatments, as I had been led to understand, or some bashing of Western medicine. She told me that the oncologist had talked her through the options for treatment in some detail, but she had decided that she didn't like the sound of them and wanted to be helped to end her life.

This scenario is increasingly common. There has been a seismic shift of opinion with regard to decision-making in the years that I have been a doctor. When I first set out on my path in medicine, the topic of medical ethics seemed quite straightforward. The standard lecture on ethics talked of four factors. Beneficence (doing the patient good), non-maleficence (not causing the patient any harm), autonomy (the right of the patient to make their own decisions), and justice (the requirement to have equitable resources throughout society). To some extent, this was both a reflection of and a cause of a kind of paternalism in which doctors would impose their will in deciding what treatment option was the best one. We have very much moved away from this model, and paternalism has become a notion rather contemptuously dismissed as belonging to a bygone era. My view is that patients, at least some of them, valued and liked the practice of paternalism. People, particularly when frightened or unwell, do not want to be given a long list of options by the doctor and then be expected to select which is best. People under those circumstances often want to be told what to do, and nearly always, when given the choice, ask what the doctor would do if it was his or her relative they were treating.

When I was a very junior doctor, I worked for a surgeon who typified everything that a man on the street thinks a surgeon is like. He was loud, opinionated, impatient, and irascible. I remember once we were doing the morning ward round, in which the consultant, surrounded by the retinue of junior doctors, nurses, physiotherapists, occupational therapists, and medical students, would sweep through the ward visiting the preoperative patients for that day's operating list, and the postoperative patients recovering from their surgery the day before. He stopped imperiously by the bedside of a middle-aged woman and explained that he would be performing her bowel surgery that day.

"What operation are you going to do, Doctor?" quavered the patient from her bed.

The surgeon flushed, affronted by the temerity of the patient in wanting to know about her operation. "Madam," he roared. The thin curtain around the bedside billowed with the force of his words. "*I* am the doctor, and *you* are the patient. I think it's best if *I* decide what operation you need." Without waiting for a reply, he flounced out of the curtained area, visibly angered, and on to the next bed, with all of us scuttling along behind to catch him up.

At the end of the ward round, the registrar, senior house officer, and I went back to the patient's bedside to apologize for the consultant's behavior, something by then we were all used to doing. As we approached, she sat up, and my registrar sat on the corner of the bed. Before he could start his apology, she gazed wistfully at the back of the consultant as he left the ward. "Ooh, what a wonderful man," she said. The apology now unnecessary, the registrar just filled her in on the timing of the surgery, and we left the ward together a few minutes later in silence.

Medical paternalism was a model and a behavior of its time. Yet in our rush to dismiss it as a relic of the past, it has been condemned as symptomatic of know-it-all doctors, and we have lost an important element of medical care, which is that patients sometimes like to have their doctor take charge, without burdening them with decisions. That era has gradually passed and been replaced by one in which patient autonomy is the value that is placed higher than all the others. This is of course apparent in our wider society, and generally it is a good thing. Yet it leads to some paradoxical ethical situations. For example, if a patient takes an overdose, and they are judged to have mental capacity—to be able to make their own decisions—or to have put in place a valid advance directive, then their right to make an autonomous decision means that a doctor trying to save them could be seen as doing them harm (and breaching the ethical duty of non-maleficence), while letting them die may be seen as doing them good (the duty of beneficence).

This leads us to one of the biggest current ethical challenges in medicine—namely the debate around assisted dying. Assisted dying means the patient ends their life with the help of a doctor. It is not the same as withdrawing life-sustaining treatment, or euthanasia, where the doctor administers the lethal medication. In assisted dying, the doctor assesses the patient, decides they are suffering and competent to make the decision to end their lives, and hands them the means to die. It is now legal in several states in the United States, some parts of Australia and Colombia, and European countries including the Netherlands, Belgium, and Switzerland. The tide is firmly set in this direction worldwide. In the UK, attempts have been made to introduce such a bill, and in my view, it is only a question of time before assisted dying becomes legal.

I will put my cards on the table and say that I am against assisted dying and most definitely against doctors being involved. While some may have made a calm and rational choice to end their lives, an unquantifiable number of people may be pressured or coerced into doing so. I remember once hearing someone say that the reason for locking your front door at night is not to prevent someone from trying to break in but to stop someone walking by from simply opening the door. Similarly, the laws against assisted dying in the UK are in place to protect the vulnerable—those who may be coerced into agreeing to end their lives so as "not to be a nuisance" to their families—not for those people who may have taken a more considered decision to end their life. As they approach the end of their lives, people feeling unwell and scared can experience a pressure, spoken or implied, to let their families collect the inheritance that they would otherwise not get if they had to pay for medical or nursing home fees. Similarly they may feel a pressure to release their families from the burden of caring for them. Vulnerable, frightened patients may feel loved, accepted, and valued by their families only if they take the decision to end their lives by assisted suicide.

Working in casualty during the Christmas holidays as a junior doctor, I remember seeing an elderly woman brought in by her son and daughter-in-law. Her son told me, "She just isn't right," and left me to get on with the assessment. I started to take the history from this lady, now in a hospital gown and sitting in the bed in a casualty bay.

"I heard you're not feeling yourself," I began.

"There's nothing wrong with me at all," she replied, starting to tear up.

"Well, your son thinks there is. Otherwise why did he bring you to casualty?"

"They just don't want me over Christmas."

I was momentarily stunned. A medical interview has its own formulaic way of assessing a problem, and I had been knocked off script. I excused myself and went to find her son and daughter-in-law to get some more detail. I was told they had left the department. I called the number for them in the notes, but the phone was switched off—they were uncontactable. I went back to the casualty area and asked the casualty sister what to do.

"Oh, granny dumping. Happens every Christmas," she said breezily, getting a vial of saline out of the cupboard.

"Well, it's the twenty-fourth of December. What am I meant to do?"

"Try social services."

I called the number and got an automated message saying that the office was now closed. Patients were starting to stack up in the casualty department as I phoned around. Eventually I realized it was hopeless, and the elderly lady was admitted to the old age ward until a solution could be found. She spent her Christmas on the ward.

That it happened at all troubled me. But that the nurses were so used to this sort of behavior that it had a name was shocking. Medicine makes you grow up fast, and I was quickly disabused of my notion that people always behave honorably or have respect for the elderly. It is at the forefront of my mind when there are discussions about assisted dying.

When these matters come before lawmakers, we are told not to worry, that there will be safeguards, and that individuals wanting to end their lives will be assessed by an experienced doctor, to ensure the vulnerable are protected. I can only say that speaking as the experienced expert who would be asked to undertake such assessments, I find this no reassurance whatsoever. It is extremely difficult to truly know someone's motives, including the motives in someone's asking for assisted dying. This is particularly the case where the individual concerned is frightened, vulnerable, or desirous of pleasing others, doing what he believes they want him to. The problem of making an accurate assessment is compounded if some doctors decide on moral grounds that they do not want to be part of assisted dying and behave as conscientious objectors. This then leaves the field open to those doctors broadly supportive of assisted dying, who may feel that the patient's wishes are understandable ("Wouldn't anyone feel like that in their position?") and so be more inclined to accede to such a request.

Indeed, there is gathering evidence that this is already the case. Assisted dying, however contentious, was originally for people with terminal illness (usually considered to be less than six months of life) who are suffering greatly. This has been expanded to include patients with psychiatric disorders who are not terminally ill in Belgium, Luxembourg, and the Netherlands, and it is estimated that now 3 percent of Belgian and Dutch assisted deaths are for psychiatric disorder. Psychiatric illness is not usually terminal, and suicidal impulses are often part of the illness itself. To have a state-sanctioned way for such people to end their lives should be a cause of concern for everyone.

One study showed that 50 percent of Dutch psychiatric patients asking to die had a personality disorder (a very unstable diagnosis with symptoms sensitive to social pressures), a figure similar to that in Belgium. Some 20 percent had never been hospitalized because of mental health problems (which called into question how severe they are), and in 56 percent of cases, loneliness and social isolation were thought to be important factors. This in turn raises the question as to whether assisted suicide is being used instead of proper social and mental health care. Perhaps the most troubling statistic in the study was that in 12 percent of such cases in the Netherlands, the three assessors had not agreed unanimously on the decision, and yet the assisted death went ahead anyway.

There is no doubt that the general public are largely in favor of assisted dying, estimated at some 80 percent of the population. What is interesting, though, is that the more information people have, the less likely they are to think that assisted dying is a good idea. A smaller percentage of doctors (figures vary from 40 to 55 percent) support the idea of assisted dying than the general public. Of those doctors working in palliative care or in elderly care, support for assisted dying is even lower. Palliative care physicians understand that for a great majority of people, good-quality palliative care means that the desire for death does diminish. My experience has been that when people are asking to die, they are commonly communicating something different. They are asking for help to live. They are saying that they can't see how they can cope with their problems and are asking for help in finding a way through the seemingly impossible difficulties that lie ahead. To take their request at face value, whisking them over to the nearest assisted dying clinic, is to abrogate our responsibilities to the patient. Assisted dying would soon become a cheaper way to treat patients, and it would be far easier to give up on people once the going gets tough. In fact, being "euthanized" is a fear that some patients do have when they come to the hospital ward, a concern that would undoubtedly worsen if this became legal.

When people are asked to imagine a future in which, say, they have been paralyzed or significantly disabled, they will commonly say that they would want to die. Some say that if they could no longer ride a bike or run or play tennis or drive, then they would prefer death to a life like that. What has become clear to me, though, is that when people are in that position—say, as a result of an accident or illness—they do not think about life (and death) in the same way anymore. When they are asked if they want to die, people are far less likely to want to be dead than they imagined they would have been. People will often find different sources of meaning in their life to match the modified circumstances that they are in.

For many, the desire for death and the request for assisted dying relate to worries about loss of control, to fears of dying in pain, and the desire not to burden others. They may consider it better to relinquish their life than to potentially relinquish their control over other things. Often this comes from a deep commitment to self-reliance, whereby they have always believed that others will let you down, a view commonly stemming from their earlier experiences in life. By contrast, some other people feel so helpless and dependent that they desire to die simply because they feel unable to cope. All of this suggests that better understanding, compassion, care, and time may be needed for our patients, and will be of help to them far more than assisted dying is. Doctors who work in palliative care are all about delivering patient choice and control in a patient's final days, and they have a much greater understanding of patient needs, which is why so many more of them are against assisted dying.

But April was sitting in front of me, asking for help to die. She said she was not talking about dying now, but soon, particularly when she could no longer live with her symptoms. She wanted me to support her in ending her life, even if it meant her going to a clinic in Switzerland. This presented a problem. According to UK guidance, we are not allowed to do anything that could be seen as encouraging, assisting, or facilitating patients who want an assisted suicide. She and I talked some more, but it was difficult to see what else I could do.

I found it hard to disentangle myself emotionally from the situation. She was someone whom I understood, indeed had come to like, but whose position, while coherent, was not one that I was able to support. We talked about whether she would consider taking the treatments recommended by the oncologists, but she was set against it. She knew I couldn't help her with assisted suicide, and we reached something of an impasse. There was no mental illness that I could diagnose, no disorder of the mind or brain—in short, nothing that was going to affect her capacity to make her own choices in life.

I lingered for a moment in the small dayroom at the end of the oncology ward. She looked wistful and said that I had surprised her, that her decision for a moment had sat less comfortably. I think she sensed that somehow her decision mattered to me, and in that respect she would have been absolutely correct. April was one of those cases where

I found it hard to separate my professional role from my personal opinions. I wanted to spend more time with her, to try to persuade her to take treatment and give herself the chance of life. But her mind was made up, and as I turned to go, leaving her on the floral-patterned sofa in the dayroom, with a plastic vase and fake flowers on a table next to it, I did so with a heavy heart. A few months later I heard she had died on the hospital ward, having been admitted the previous week. I have no idea whether she tried to get into an assisted suicide clinic, but I know she didn't end up there. I do hope, however, that when the end came, she had peace of mind.

THE PRICE OF
A TROUBLED MIND

K aren came into my consulting room during one afternoon clinic.
I was finishing off a slew of emails, which had been building up
over the past several days and which exuded the feeble menace of unfinished work. Most emails were circulars, which got deleted straightaway. Some needed a brief reply, which they got, and one or two emails
merited a bit more thought, so I put them to one side. There was an
email from Luiz, a fellow psychiatrist. For reasons long forgotten, our
email exchanges have adopted the language of Soviet-era Politburo
members, probably subconsciously stemming from the feeling that the
NHS behaves as a kind of badly run totalitarian state. I had asked him
to sponsor me for a half marathon that I was running on behalf of a
medical charity. "Comrade Santhouse," the email began, "I suggested
to the junior members of the local committee that they should each
make a voluntary contribution of 3 roubles and 25 kopecks. Young
people have ideals and can do very well without potatoes for a week.
They all democratically and enthusiastically supported the motion. The
girls of our Sunshine Movement have already started to organize the

Victory Banquet in your honor (at the Lubyanka People's canteen, just in case you don't complete the race)." There was a sponsorship receipt from him. I laughed and began to compose a reply when the receptionist rang to let me know the first patient of that afternoon's clinic had arrived.

I rummaged around on my desk and found the notes and referral letter. It was from one of the consultants in diabetes and endocrinology. Karen was forty-nine, with three children, and her diabetes control had been consistently poor over the years. She had already begun to develop complications, including impairment of her kidney function, as well as some eye problems for which she had recently been referred for laser treatment. The consultant and her team had tried all different sorts of insulin preparations, routes and timings of administration, yet to no avail. Karen's diabetic control continued to deteriorate. Each day of poor control was, in tiny increments, leading to a steadily worsening outcome. There was a note of exasperation in the referral letter ("We have tried everything . . . despite all our warnings, Karen refuses to . . ."). A psychiatry referral must have been the last roll of the dice for the diabetes team, a final attempt to salvage a reasonable outcome from a deteriorating situation ("We wondered if a psychiatric assessment might be able to offer a way forward"). The diabetic team's exasperation reflected the helplessness doctors feel watching a patient's health deteriorate, made worse by the fact that the patient is able to change the outcome, if only they chose to. We have all been in similar situations. We have all watched bright children coast along, impervious to the pleas of teachers and parents that they could really excel, if only they wanted to. Football academies are full of talented players who never realize their talent because they lack the drive and drift down to the lower leagues. And in medicine, there is nothing quite as heartbreaking as watching an entirely avoidable tragedy unfold.

Karen was not tight-lipped and defiant as I had imagined her. I have had people come to my clinics before under pressure, determined to declare it a waste of time and intent on playing each question with a dead hand. Karen, though, seemed at ease. She looked younger than her years, her hair straight and shoulder-length, and she was wearing outdoor clothes: navy blue all-weather trousers and a dark blue fleece. She had worked on the railways since leaving school. She had two sons and a daughter, and a husband for whom she had little regard. There was no open hostility toward him, but rather a contemptuous indifference. He loved her, but she simply saw this as further evidence that he was needy and weak.

Karen could not remember a time that she had not had type 1 diabetes. It had been diagnosed during her childhood and had colored her memories of growing up. She was always the child who had to watch what she ate and had to inject herself with insulin before meals, which she found embarrassing. As her teenage years progressed, she increasingly resented the restrictions that having diabetes placed on her life. She had to check her blood sugar reading regularly, before each meal, and she began to see life ahead of her as full of burden and restriction, which other people did not have to share.

She married in her late teens to a childhood sweetheart. It was an infatuation that did not last. She began to scorn his lack of ambition and soon tired of the life she was living with him. It felt as if the net was closing in, her diabetes and her humdrum life trapping her. Her job was the only thing she enjoyed, taking some pleasure in the freedom of working outdoors. "I wouldn't want your job," she said to me, "being stuck in an office all day."

She tried hard to fit in at work and enjoyed the camaraderie of her colleagues. As she was out for most of her day, she ate lunch on the go and was too self-conscious to inject with insulin. She didn't want her work colleagues to know that she had diabetes, and anyway she could never find a quiet spot to inject.

"Do you think they would have minded?" I asked. "I mean, knowing you had diabetes."

She looked at me with disdain, sighed. I wasn't getting it. "I just want to be normal. Not to have to think about it every day."

It was like a late adolescence. She began to neglect her diabetes and found it easier not to check her blood sugars, because then she didn't have a problem. She stayed late for afterwork drinks, and for the first time enjoyed being carefree. Gradually, silently, diabetic complications started to accumulate. She started missing outpatient appointments, because she saw the hospital's advice as nagging, and in any case she felt fine. Over time, the poorly controlled diabetes began to affect her kidney function. Rather than motivate her, the realization that she had developed complications worsened things. It was hard for her to explain, but it seemed to come down to this: If she couldn't be completely well, she didn't want to be well at all. And now that she had allowed her health to be affected, it was all too late.

A part of me could understand what she had said, despite the confused logic behind it. I had experienced a trivial but surprisingly irritating moment a couple of weeks before. By chance, a friend mentioned they were flying to Rome free on frequent-flier miles. A conversation ensued about how the whole air mile thing worked. It wasn't long before I realized that if only I had gotten a credit card with air miles, I could have had enough points by then for flights to anywhere in the world. The thought needled me. Getting the air miles credit card now would only remind me of what I should have done years before, and it seemed easier not to get one, and not to think about it anymore. I constructed reasons it probably wasn't worth it. Any logical analysis would have demonstrated that my position was against my own interests. It wasn't too late, after all. I wasn't that old. Why not just start now? Yet I've long since come to realize that many decisions we make, even important ones, are driven by emotion and have little to do with rationality.

I asked Karen what had made her come to see me. She had still not really warmed up to the consultation. She thought for a moment. I could see her weighing up whether she was going to tell me.

"It was the eyes," she said. "Going blind frightens me."

She didn't care too much about dying, but living without being able to see, without being able to do a job that she enjoyed, was to her a fate worse than death. She just didn't know how to turn things around. She felt defeated by her situation, angry with herself for letting it get this far, and miserable every day. She found it increasingly hard to get out of bed each morning, lacking the will to do many of the household tasks that needed doing. Her husband was trying his best, but she had little time for him. The thought of how her children were managing made her feel even more guilty. When the doctors asked her to think of her children— to take her insulin for them, if not for herself—it was too much to bear. She resented her children being used in this way, although she knew the doctors had a point. She had gotten caught in a sinkhole of her own making, and to continue dropping into it felt easier than pulling herself clear. She presented a mixture of helplessness and defiance, and the defiance made helping her much harder.

It should have been so straightforward. Diabetes is a disease that, even if it is not curable, is manageable. We have the medical expertise to guide treatment, and we have the medicines available, at no cost to the patient in the UK. The consequences of poorly controlled diabetes are considerable, threatening eyesight, kidneys, nerves, feet, and the cardiovascular system. Yet despite the hospital's significant investment in her care, Karen's unwillingness to manage her diabetes was leading to treatment failure and avoidable, costly complications.

From a psychiatry perspective, Karen was in that diagnostic gray area that all psychiatrists—in fact, all doctors—have to get comfortable inhabiting. She had symptoms of depression, but a diagnosis of depression did not capture all of her problems. Depression did not explain the defiance, the anger, and the sense of grievance and injustice that she felt. More important, though, even if the depression was clear-cut, I was sure that Karen would see the prescription of antidepressants as a reflexive, unthinking response, and I couldn't see much good coming from me suggesting them.

In fact, Karen had had enough of being told what to do. I decided to let her make all the suggestions as to what to do next in order to take back some control over her life. As I said, there was something adolescent about her behavior, and I reckoned that being treated like a grown-up, rather than infantilized by the medical system, would be a good start. I asked her what she thought would happen if she carried on the way things had been going. She didn't need long to think.

"Blind, probably. Out of a job."

There was a pause. I put the question the other way around. "Well, where do you think you'd be in a few years' time if you managed to take the treatment that the diabetes team recommend?"

"Probably doing the same as I am now. Working, seeing my friends, the usual."

The choice was obvious, but I wasn't going to suggest it. There was another silence.

"But you're not sure what you're going to do." It was a statement rather than a question. The defiance gave way to tears, now that I hadn't given her anything to react against.

"I don't think I can. I just don't know." She looked agitated, a reflection of her unresolved internal discomfort. Was she going to let her anger and her misery destroy her? Or was she going to choose to live, but in a way that she saw as a capitulation? The choice may have been clear to me, but it was not to her.

Patients like Karen are undoubtedly suffering, trapped in indecision, their physical health slowly deteriorating. Yet there is a financial cost to the psychological difficulties, aside from the personal cost. The gathering complications, which for Karen included the looming threat of kidney failure, dialysis, and blindness, all add up to a significant expenditure in medical care. Added to that are the economic costs of her losing her job, her income, and her disability benefits. However Karen's symptoms could be conceptualized, maybe as depression or perhaps more simply as something about her personality and way of thinking about her illness, the outcome to the wider health economy is much the same.

Scaling that up to the whole of the UK, the King's Fund report estimated that individuals with long-term conditions are two to three times more likely to have mental health problems than the rest of the population. Even if we put aside the reduced quality of life, it costs the UK economy an estimated £8 to £13 billion extra per year. In the United States, a study examining over 600,000 insurance claims showed the average additional cost in depressed patients with medical problems was from over $1,500 to just over $15,000 per patient, depending on the condition being looked at. It is a similar story throughout the West. A German study of over 300,000 patients showed that psychiatric illness increased medical inpatient hospital costs by 40 percent, an enormous cost to any healthcare system.

Many other studies have explored the effects of depression on long-term health outcomes. The results are predictably grim. In pretty much any illness you care to mention, depression will have a significant negative impact. For example, depression worsens the outcome after a stroke. It results in increased disability, as well as cognitive impairment and increased chances of dying. Yet despite the fact that this phenomenon is well described in the medical literature, the treatment of depression after a stroke is not given the same priority as physical treatments, such as clot-busting drugs and physiotherapy.

We know the same is true of depression and heart disease. Depression itself is a significant risk factor for developing heart disease. And after a heart attack, the presence of depression makes prolonged illness and death more likely. It is probable that this happens through a combination of the chemical changes caused by depression, but perhaps even more important, through the effects of depression on the morale of the individual. Depressed people take less care of themselves. They may, for example, carry on smoking, or continue with a generally unhealthy, sedentary lifestyle and diet, or lack the motivation to attend follow-up appointments. Again, all of these possibilities are well known, but the emphasis on the treatment of depression in the context of cardiac disease gets nothing like the same level of attention as the use of cardiac drugs. It is an odd paradox that makes little sense. We have a treatable illness, depression, and we know that treating it will make a difference to overall illness and survival. So why does depression get a lower billing? I believe there are two main reasons. The first is because there is a prevailing attitude that depression is "understandable." It is seen by many people, including doctors, as a normal reaction ("Wouldn't anyone feel like that in their position?"). The second reason is that medicine has become increasingly atomized into subspecialties, and cardiologists generally feel comfortable with the heart, but far less confident when it comes to treating (or even recognizing) disorders of the mind.

You could walk around the different departments in any hospital, as I do each day, and in each hospital department you would find a similar story. Patients with diseases of the airways, if they develop depression, have poorer survival rates and experience more symptoms. They are less likely to give up smoking (itself usually a major reason why they were in a chest clinic in the first place). Similarly, people with diabetes who develop depression are less careful about administering their medication (diabetic medication and insulin injections can be quite complicated to manage). They are less likely to stick to a diabetic diet, more likely to develop eye disease, and more likely to develop nerve damage as well as other complications of their diabetes; they also have higher overall healthcare costs than nondepressed people with diabetes. Overall, if you have a medical illness like diabetes, having depression is likely to increase your risk of illness and death.

The emphasis given to psychiatry in general hospitals doesn't even come close to reflecting the extent of the problem that illnesses like depression cause. Depression is not an add-on to a long-term physical illness, something that can either be treated or safely ignored, depending on whether anyone has noticed it or has the time and interest to treat it. Rather, depression is usually at the very center of why people will take their medications or not, decide to make lifestyle changes or not. And even worse, there is something about depression itself that seems to be toxic to the body, that leads to people dying younger, with studies consistently showing a higher death rate among depressed people than nondepressed individuals of the same age. Yet the provision of psychiatry in most general hospitals ranges from almost nonexistent to inadequate, and where psychiatry in the general hospital exists at all, it is usually in Accident and Emergency, with an emphasis on self-harm and attempted suicide.

I saw Karen several times over the months afterward. Her diabetic control did not change. I felt irritated, goaded even, by her lack of progress. I was frustrated and was getting drawn into the experience of the diabetes team when they referred her, watching helplessly as her health slowly deteriorated, her kidney function worsening and her eyesight progressively compromised. I wondered why she kept coming back when she seemed to be making no progress and expending no effort. I ruminated on this and came up with two answers. The first was that if Karen found the appointments a waste of time, she wouldn't have kept coming back, so she must have been getting something out of them. My second thought was that the way I felt was probably a fair reflection of what Karen was feeling—powerless, frustrated, helpless, worried. It has been my experience that the way a patient makes you feel is usually communicating something, even though it is nonverbal and indirect. I put that to her, identifying the emotions. It seemed to introduce more honesty into our discussion, and she was able to talk more about being trapped by her circumstances, frightened, unsure what to do.

I asked her what she saw as the major difficulties in following the advice of the diabetic team, and she spoke again of the fact that she didn't want her work colleagues to know about her diabetes and that she didn't want her life to have to change. I was still careful not to offer any suggestions, since she was going to find it easier to follow her own advice than mine. The discussions followed the principles of what is known as motivational interviewing, where you encourage the patient themselves to identify solutions to their own problems, guiding them to the destination they are trying to reach, but not telling them what to do.

She wanted her workmates to know about her diabetes, but for it then not to be discussed so she could take her insulin without any awkwardness. We gradually advanced. She decided to start by telling a work friend about her diabetes, the person she was closest to at work. It had taken her weeks to build up to this point. I asked her what had happened.

"Her husband's got diabetes. And she knew anyway. She's seen the blood monitoring kit in my locker."

I tried to nod supportively, in the manner of a psychiatrist not judging anyone, but instead snorted with laughter. "After all that!" I said. "Did it . . ." I was about to ask a question, but the pathos and comedy of the human condition had eclipsed it, and I laughed until tears came to my eyes. I felt a great sympathy for us as human beings, caught up in our inner worlds of such resolute importance and iron rules, only to discover that they do not withstand the faintest contact with the real world. It was sad and it was funny, and Karen, despite herself, was laughing, too.

Progress was quicker from there, and Karen's mood noticeably improved over the subsequent weeks. Insurmountable problems, once she broke them down, proved to be manageable, and she increasingly realized that all the barriers to progressing with her life existed only in her own mind. She had begun to monitor her blood glucose and take her insulin more reliably. She had also started to reconcile herself to the damage she had done to her kidneys and eyes and resolved to at least not make it worse. I discharged her soon afterward. Although her life was not straightforward, and there were differences with her husband that did not portend well, she could at least make decisions less encumbered by her low mood and sense of hopelessness.

The sad truth, though, is that psychological difficulties rarely get much attention and are even less likely to get effective treatment. Maybe this is because treatments are not in the form of the latest medication, directed against a newly discovered chemical and released with fanfare by a pharmaceutical company. Psychiatric treatment can be difficult and needs specialist knowledge and expertise. There are relatively few psychiatrists who specialize in the interface between the physical and psychological, or the psychiatric consequences of long-term conditions. When there's no psychiatrist or psychologist available, it can be easier just not to look for the psychological problems. The doctor is more likely to apply the treatment that is readily available, following the old adage that when your only tool is a hammer, you turn every problem into a nail.

Sometimes it feels that treating one patient at a time in my clinic is a hopeless task, yet there is a reason why there are so few psychiatrists in the area, which is that there are so few hospitals prepared to pay for them. Despite lots of discussion about the parity of physical and mental health, the reality is a million miles from the rhetoric.

CAPACITY

It was my very first month as a consultant psychiatrist. Being appointed as consultant was a process that had taken me eighteen years to reach since I had first entered medical school. Over that time I had sat for more exams than I could count. (In fact I once tried, but gave up after forty.) I had taken my last exam a few months before my thirtieth birthday. Even after the exams were complete, there were several more years of training. At this point I was now in my mid-thirties, and although I felt ready for the job, nothing quite prepares you for taking final responsibility for all of the clinical as well as management problems. I was still finding my feet, getting to know colleagues and putting up in my new office all the pictures that I wasn't allowed to put on the walls at home. There was an anemic-looking watercolor of my old Cambridge college, Emmanuel, a graduation present from my parents; a photograph of me at age twenty-one with my college football team, my bouffant hairstyle rising vertically upward from my head; a kind of abstract drawing bought for me by friends for my eighteenth birthday; and a framed share certificate for Manchester City Football Club, another birthday present. My office was on the ground floor, with an internal view of the hospital atrium and walkways. It had no natural light, except for outside my office, several floors above, where there was a skylight. For two weeks in June, when the path of the sun was just right, direct sunlight would angle into my office through the skylight for an hour in the day. The contrast with the rest of the year's oppressive gloom was so stark that paradoxically the bright beam of sunlight made me miserable.

My remit was to build up the psychiatry service in the general hospital, delivering a psychiatry service to the medical and surgical teams. I spent my first month unpacking boxes and answering a flood of emails from occupational health, so it was a relief to take a call from one of the kidney consultants. He wanted me to see Dom, a twenty-six-year-old man who had developed kidney failure quite suddenly the previous month. Unlike many of their patients, for whom kidney failure is a gradual process, Dom was what they referred to as a "crash lander." Most patients with failing kidneys have time, often years, to acclimatize to the steady progression of their kidney failure and to discuss dialysis options or the possibility of a transplant with their team. Dom, however, had been brought into casualty in a state of collapse. He was given emergency dialysis, stabilized, and then sent home after a ten-day admission, to continue dialysis as an outpatient.

This was a month ago. Since then, he had been coming to the hospital for dialysis three times per week, on Mondays, Wednesdays, and Fridays. The day I was asked to see him, he had arrived as usual for his dialysis. It was a little unclear what had happened next, but the upshot was he had made up his mind to stop dialysis. He had refused to be connected to the dialysis machine and had become confrontational with the nursing staff, so security had been called. In my experience, there are few situations in hospital that can't be made worse by the arrival of security. The renal team were unsure what to do. What they were more certain about was that if Dom continued to refuse dialysis, he would very likely be dead within a week. Dom, however, did not feel he needed to see a psychiatrist and had required some persuading to see me. On the way over to see him, I felt uneasy. The situation was time-pressured, dangerous, and fraught with uncertainty.

Wearing jeans and a black shirt, Dom was in the waiting room of the outpatient department. He had a coarse round face and a scratchy full-face beard. A tattoo stretched from somewhere beneath his T-shirt, radiating to his neck. It looked like a bird's wing, but perhaps it was a leaf or petal. As I approached him, I noticed two security guards hovered in the background, unsure what they should be doing. Dom radiated boredom and a simmering impatience. Even as we walked into one of the clinic rooms, he was quick to let me know he had had enough of waiting around and wanted to go home. He told me that this was a waste of time, and nothing was going to change his mind.

I motioned for him to sit down. "Well, since you've waited all this time to talk to me, what did you want to talk about?" I asked.

He looked wrong-footed, momentarily confused. "I told you. I didn't want to talk to you."

"Oh, I was under the impression you did. And me, a trained psychiatrist. How did I misread the signs?"

Dom laughed, and although the mask was quickly put back in place, the tension had eased. He turned a little more toward me and began to talk about the experience of recent weeks. The doctors weren't certain why his kidneys had suddenly failed, although the damage was now irreversible. He told me that he still lived at home. He didn't have a job, although he was able to make money through various enterprises that were not, if I understood his meaning correctly, entirely legitimate.

His life was lived in a haphazard sort of a way. He had been expelled from two different schools—once after he was caught trying to break into a teacher's car, and the second time for taking drugs on school premises. He seemed to lack a sense of identity, uncertain about what he stood for. He found his enjoyment through drugs and brief, intense, but shallow relationships. His relationships were always over within weeks, his love a mile wide but an inch deep. At times of crisis, he would struggle to cope with his inner tension and generally found relief through cutting himself. This was usually with scissors or a razor blade. At other times, he would stick pins in his skin, and occasionally he burned himself with a cigarette. He found the pain and the sight of blood cathartic. As he told me this, he rolled up his sleeve to reveal dozens of scars, some old and white, others redder and more recent.

The decision to stop his dialysis had come to him that morning. After an argument with his mother, he decided that he had had enough of life.

"What did you argue about?"

"She was on at me again about getting a job. She doesn't want me at home. I told her, 'If you hate me that much, why don't you just say it outright?'"

"Perhaps she cares about you, which is why she takes an interest in what you're doing."

He shook his head emphatically. There was no willingness to concede anything. He got up to leave.

"So what's going to happen with the dialysis?" I asked him.

"I'm going home, and you can't stop me. My mum's waiting for me."

"Your mother? Waiting where?"

"In the *waiting* room," he said, rolling his eyes.

I had seen a woman next to him on the way in, sitting with a straight back, fawn coat buttoned to her chin. She looked prim, conventional, anxious.

"That was your mother? In the brown coat?" I had assumed she was another patient. She looked nothing like him, particularly in her demeanor. "Do you mind if I talk to her?"

I went to the waiting room, where she was sitting on the edge of the seat, staring at the door as I exited the clinic room. She leaped up, her face creased with concern, dark rings under her eyes. She was keen to talk, so I motioned toward a quiet area near the nurses' room. Now that we were alone, though, she was suddenly silent, uncertain how to start. The void created by her silence made me think of a line by Samuel Daniel, the sixteenth-century poet: "Striving to tell his woes, words would not come; for light cares speak, when mighty griefs are dumb." Dom, it turned out, had been a mighty grief to her. "He's never given me a second's happiness since the day he was born," she began, a statement shocking both in its bluntness and the sincerity with which she said it. She had three children, and he was the middle one. From as far back as she could remember, he had been getting into trouble at school and found it hard to make friends. Academically he was average but put little effort into his studies and was not popular with his teachers. She told me Dom had always been a risk-taker, but in an impulsive and reckless rather than a calculated way. His brother and his sister barely spoke to him. She felt a maternal love for him, dutiful, correct, but nothing more. Now she was facing his death, and all her feelings of regret, remorse, and anguish came flooding to the surface.

By then, based on what I had read in his notes, and what both Dom and his mother had told me, this was an issue of personality rather than mental illness. Psychiatry has always had an uneasy relationship with personality disorders. There is little consistency in the way such disorders are diagnosed, even though there are rules for diagnosing them. There are many different subtypes of personality disorder, but they all have a common factor. They create difficulties for the person suffering with them in getting on in life. Personality disorders make it hard for people to form the relationships they need to hold down jobs, or to develop romantic relationships and friendships. Impulsive or disruptive behaviors, self-harm, and brushes with the law are all far more common among people with personality disorders. And because of the difficulties in diagnosing personality disorders, there is good evidence that these labels are given to people who doctors just don't like. If a patient is difficult, rude, or troublesome, doctors can easily forget that such behaviors may be because the patient is frightened or upset and attribute the behavior not to the situation but to the patient's personality. For this reason, I am usually wary of making a diagnosis like this without good evidence, and rarely after a first meeting. I am also fairly reluctant to make a diagnosis of personality disorder for another reason, which is that it feels like an attack on the person's very soul, the essence of who they are, to say that their personality is "disordered." Yet all the evidence so far pointed in that direction for Dom.

There is another reason why psychiatrists find dealing with personality disorders difficult, and that is because treatments for them are generally unimpressive. If personalities are fixed and stable, then the concept of "illness" and "treatment" doesn't really make sense. Where there is improvement, the time course for any changes is usually measured in years. In short, there seemed little that would change Dom's attitude or his view of his situation. Dom was going to leave the department and go home to die. It was with a sinking heart that I went back to see him.

The problem was that I didn't really think Dom wanted to die. Yet if I was going to make him have treatment against his wishes, I had to establish that he lacked mental capacity to make the decision, because that was the only way I could legally compel him to have treatment. To show that someone lacks capacity, you need to answer a series of questions. So first, did Dom have a disorder of the mind or brain? Well, not exactly. I suppose you could make an argument that personality disorders are disorders of the mind, but aren't they really just a different way of seeing and interacting with the world? Don't we all have differing personalities and world views? We vote differently and respond to criticism differently; we have different levels of tolerance to frustration. These are not disorders of the mind in the way that, say, schizophrenia is.

I moved on to the next question. Did he understand the procedure (in this case dialysis) and understand the risks of refusing it as opposed to the risks and benefits of having it? Well, he knew very well that refusing dialysis would lead to his death over the next few days, so that had to be a yes. Finally, could he balance the pros and cons of either accepting or rejecting the dialysis to arrive at a decision? As always in psychiatry, this question was where the real difficulties lay. We are emotional creatures who factor in dozens of issues when we make decisions, and often make them emotionally, rather than rationally. To what extent is a decision to die rather than to live ever rational? How can we tell whether the decision to choose death is a reflection of mental illness or of personality in cases like these? And, circling back to where we started, to what extent is a personality disorder a mental illness in any case?

Dom was adamant. He was going home, and nobody could stop him. He didn't want to live anymore, and that was that. Reluctantly and with considerable unease, I agreed that he could make that choice if he wanted to.

It's not often I leave work with a case still lingering in my mind. Over the course of an average week I make a number of decisions, hear a great number of patient stories, and am exposed to the range of emotional pain that people suffer. I do get it, but I don't feel the emotions that the patient feels. It would be hard to do my job otherwise. But I was worried, and anxiety about a patient is different from empathy, because really it was an anxiety about myself as well. I wasn't sure I had made the right decision.

I couldn't settle that evening. Eventually I decided to watch a film to take my mind off things, but it was hopeless. I kept having to press pause so that I could worry a little bit more, and I eventually tired of the film. My worrying was like having a bit of orange stuck between my teeth that my tongue kept going back to. Even when I was distracted for a while, I had a sense of foreboding. I would sit uneasily for a bit until I remembered what was causing it and then would pick over it some more. The image of Dom and his mother leaving the department, with his mother, a head shorter than him, shoulders bowed, heaving with sobs, was haunting me.

I arrived at my office the next morning and started to work through my emails. There was one from Luiz. With all that had been going on the day before, I had forgotten to attend the hospital's mandatory training event. "Comrade Santhouse," it began. "The Committee noted your absence at the Hospital Trust's vibrant and inspirational mandatory training. I myself, who set the example of sensitivity to equality and diversity to all, under the motherly wings of our beloved Party, still attended the Equality and Diversity training. You may have forgotten that I was awarded the Medal of the Most Sensitive Comrade by the Presidium itself, but now my sensitivity for Comrade Santhouse is no more. I hope Comrade S appreciates that this little vignette holds valuable lessons for us all." Laughing, I booked myself on the next mandatory training day, put it in my diary, and carried on working through my emails. There was an email from the dialysis consultant to say that Dom had changed his mind that same evening, come back to the hospital, and had his dialysis. I shook my head in relief and exasperation. The email asked what I had said to him to change his mind. I doubted it was anything I had done. But with a sense of relief and goodwill to all, I set about my morning clinic.

Capacity decisions are an increasing source of referrals in general hospital psychiatry. Getting treatment is not just about whether there is treatment available, but whether someone chooses to have it. The reasons people either choose or decline treatments can be difficult to understand. Sometimes people just make unwise or irrational decisions, and that is their right. Sometimes, though, people's decision-making process is hindered by a mental health problem that can be hard to diagnose. Yet the law assumes that psychiatrists can see into people's minds, understand their workings, and make a judgment as to whether they have the capacity to make treatment decisions.

It is common for people being treated in a general hospital (not just a psychiatric hospital) to lack capacity to decide on treatment. One study showed at least 40 percent of patients admitted to a medical ward lack capacity, a problem that was rarely recognized by the clinical team. Most of the time, though, patients who aren't feeling well go along with what the doctor tells them is best, and everyone is happy. Trusting your doctor isn't the same thing as having capacity, but for most people it seems good enough. I rarely, if ever, get referred these patients, so in general hospital psychiatry we are seeing only the tip of the iceberg.

Some time after seeing Dom, I was called to one of the surgical wards, where Ray, a sixty-nine-year-old, had been brought in after being found collapsed in his nursing home by a carer. It turned out that a large prostate "the size of a grapefruit" (urologists always seem to measure prostates in relation to fruit, typically using oranges, grapefruits, or melons) had been obstructing outflow from the bladder. The resulting pressure had backed up all the way to the kidneys and had caused them to fail. The urologists had decided that the best treatment would be a fairly routine operation to remove the prostate—not without its dangers, but since this was the third time the patient had presented in exactly the same way, the alternatives didn't seem to be working.

Ray himself lived an isolated life. He had been employed for a time as a bricklayer but had not worked for many years. He was cut adrift from his family and had no friends. Talking to him, I could understand why. His conversational style was abrasive, and it was all but impossible to develop any warmth or rapport. He had a view of the world that was roughly on the border of what most people would consider "normal." He held views about UFOs and the paranormal, which he shared as though the things he was talking about were established facts, hidden from us by successive governments. Consistent with this, he saw his hospital admission as a form of oppression. No, he didn't believe there was anything wrong with his prostate. He was implacably of the view that his admission and proposed operation were for the purposes of unlicensed experimentation. He brooked no argument. He wanted to go home and be left alone. I called up his carers in the nursing home. They told me he never had visitors, and they had never met any of his family. He spent most of his time shut away in his room, and his paranoia and hostility had intensified over the past year or so. He appeared not to understand the gravity of his situation, resolutely denying anything was wrong with him. His mental illness made it impossible for him to weigh the pros and cons of treatment or lack of it. The unavoidable conclusion was that he lacked capacity to make good decisions about his own treatment.

The following lunchtime I was on the top deck of the number 40 bus, traveling to my Thursday-afternoon clinic at the Maudsley, when my mobile rang. As always, I was trying to answer emails, read and catch up on some papers, and now trying to answer the phone at the same time. It was the urology surgeon. "That patient you saw yesterday."

"Uh-huh," I said distractedly, trying to reach a piece of paper that had slipped under my seat.

"He's in theater with me now, about to operate on him."

"Good. Don't mess it up, then."

"Um, yes. I was just checking you're still okay with it."

I came to my senses and focused on the call. Actually, now that it had come to it, it did seem quite daunting, operating on a patient who was opposing the surgery, even if he wasn't actively resisting. Until then

I had always thought the difficult decision was in not treating a patient who could be helped. Now that we were undertaking lifesaving surgery on a patient who had not given his consent, even if his reasons for withholding consent were a consequence of mental illness, it felt like a huge undertaking. I could understand why the surgeon was so uneasy.

There was a surprising finale to the case. I saw Ray on the ward a week or so later, when I was reviewing another patient. I wanted to tiptoe past his bed, anticipating a very noisy and public dressing down, but he caught sight of me almost as soon as I stepped onto the ward and beckoned me over. He greeted me with something approaching warmth—certainly no rancor. I asked him how he was feeling. He was feeling easier and seemed relieved that his problems had been resolved. He was in a better frame of mind than when I had first assessed him, less stressed and agitated. It was a relief both that the surgery had worked well and that Ray bore no grudges. Not wanting to push my luck, though, when it came to exiting the ward, I took another route out.

In some ways Ray had been an easy and quick decision. The consequences of delay in situations like this can be a real problem. A couple of years later, I was asked by the dermatology team to see a man with skin cancer. Harvey was in his late fifties and had been diagnosed a few weeks prior to my meeting him. The dermatologists and oncologists had met, agreed on a treatment plan, and presented it to him. Harvey had refused. His reason for refusal was difficult to discern initially, and he didn't seem interested in talking. He answered the questions he was asked, directly and with little detail or embellishment. As he spoke to me, I was drawn into his sad and isolated world. He lived alone in a one-bedroom flat. He had some intermittent contact with relatives nearby, but no friends and nobody who particularly cared for him. He spent his days watching television, went shopping as infrequently as he could manage, and lived on cups of tea and toast. His clothes were worn through, he was thin, and his face had a lived-in look, with sallow, sunken cheeks. His beard was gray, almost white, but with brown nicotine stains from his pack-a-day smoking habit, and the fingertips between his middle and index fingers were similarly stained. He appeared far older than his years. It was difficult to form a rapport with him. Harvey steadfastly believed that he was a talented physician and had concluded that he did not have a cancer, as the doctors were trying to insist, but rather this was an infection. He said that he was prepared to take antibiotics, and this would resolve his problems to the satisfaction of everyone.

Harvey was not a doctor; in fact he had not had a job in decades. His life had been defined by relapsing schizophrenia, and the highest educational level he had achieved was school exams at age sixteen. He was far from stupid, but he was certainly not educated. I went back to his medical records and could see that his delusion of being a doctor was long-standing.

A similar case had come before the English courts some years earlier. It concerned a patient known only as C. C was diabetic and had developed gangrene in his leg. The attending surgeon advised that he needed a below-knee amputation to avoid a sepsis spreading into his bloodstream and killing him. Without an amputation, the surgeon thought that the chances of his survival were low, somewhere around 15 percent. C, who had a long-standing history of paranoid schizophrenia and was in a secure psychiatric hospital at the time this took place, refused the surgery. He had a delusional belief that he was a world-famous physician, and presumably therefore thought that he knew better. He believed that he would be cured, expressing faith in the hospital staff, although he did accept that he might die from the gangrene. The presiding judge took the view that C understood enough about the gangrene and the pros and cons of declining an operation to make his own choice to refuse the surgery. The judge did not feel his schizophrenia or his delusional beliefs were enough of an interference in his decision-making capacity about his gangrenous leg.

Although C (perhaps to the surprise of the attending doctors) recovered, I found the judgment hard to understand. Dr. Tony Zigmond, a psychiatrist and former Royal College of Psychiatrists' Lead on Mental Health Law, recounts in his book *A Clinician's Brief Guide to the Mental Health Act* an addendum to the case. C's solicitor had suggested he make a will, given the likelihood of his dying from the gangrene. C agreed to make the will but said that he wanted to leave the money to himself, since he would need it after he had died. Given that statement, I find it hard to accept that C was fully able to work through the consequences of refusing surgery; it's as if C considered death as some kind of impermanent state. The judge's decision is also difficult to understand given that C's consideration of the decision was guided by his belief in his own opinion as a surgeon, when he was nothing of the sort. That he recovered is simply good luck, rather than good judgment. It's like correctly guessing the answer to a math problem without knowing how to solve it. The case, though, illustrated the complexities of capacity decisions, and particularly of the nuances of how people weigh decisions before deciding on a course of action.

Despite the ruling in the case of C, I was of the view that Harvey lacked capacity to refuse treatment. He didn't accept the diagnosis of cancer, nor did he believe that he might die. In not even acknowledging the possibility of a fatal outcome, he was even less able than C to weigh the pros and cons of treatment. The problem here was not whether he lacked capacity, as I felt that decision was quite straightforward. The problem was that even if he did lack capacity, what were we going to do about it? It wasn't a situation like C's or Ray's, where a quick operation would resolve the matter at hand. If Harvey was going to receive chemotherapy, it would take his active cooperation, not just on one occasion, but over a sustained period of time. It just isn't realistic to administer chemotherapy to a patient refusing treatment and actively resisting. There is a danger to the staff, and it may even cause complications that hasten death.

The only option was to try to treat his schizophrenia as aggressively as possible, in the hope that an improvement in his mental health would reduce his delusional belief about being a doctor. This would allow him to acknowledge what the real doctors were telling him. It was a race against time, because for each week that went by without chemotherapy, the chances of successful treatment receded further.

Again that familiar sense of unease came over me, the feeling I only ever get with capacity cases: uncertainty and helplessness. If I'm really honest with myself, I wanted to shake Harvey until he understood, until he realized what was at stake. It was the same feeling I'd had about Dom, even though their cases were very different. Mine was a longing to do the impossible, to treat a refractory mental disorder in an impossible time frame, and for life to blossom rather than be extinguished. I appreciate that the patient is the one with the illness, but there's a part of me that suffers with these cases. Harvey's mental health never stabilized to the extent that he could receive treatment, and he eventually passed the point of no return. By then he was under the care of the community mental health team, and when I next bumped into the community psychiatrist, he told me that Harvey had died.

Dom died, too. A few months after I saw him for the first time, he once again made the decision to withdraw from dialysis. There had been several episodes in between, in which he had impulsively decided to stop and then changed his mind. Yet increasingly his wish to stop dialysis became more consistent and less impulsive, until finally he simply didn't return for treatment. His light had briefly shone and been extinguished, a victim of his own personality.

There are too many tragedies in medicine to keep up, and it's impossible to expend emotion on each one and retain your own sanity. Yet I find capacity cases uniquely poignant. There's something about them that gets under my skin. Capacity assessments highlight a flaw in the way medicine is practiced. The medical conceit is that technical advances translate into better patient outcomes. The framing is far too narrow, though. What patients are prepared to believe, what treatments they will accept—this has nothing to do with medical advances and everything to do with their psychological makeup. People will decide which symptoms to exaggerate and which to conceal. People can be irrational, stubborn, or depressed, or just have a different way of seeing things. All of these thought processes and decisions are present in every medical interaction. Some people will refuse treatment because they are angry or frightened. Some patients accept treatment without fully understanding the implications. While it is the higher-profile or contentious cases that get the media attention, many such cases are not even recognized, let alone considered. Over time I have got used to capacity assessments. I no longer lose sleep over them, but more than any other, referrals for capacity assessments still set me on edge.

FINAL DAYS

One cold but sunny winter afternoon, I was called to one of the surgical wards to see Harry, a sixty-one-year-old who had been told he was dying of an inoperable bowel cancer. I sat at his bedside as he told me about his life. He had grown up in Scotland, married at twenty-one, and remained married to the same woman for forty years. They had two adult sons, who both lived a few streets away from them, and both sons now had children of their own. Harry had worked as a window cleaner and for some time had run his own business, which made a regular and steady living. He played on the pub darts team, liked watching television, and enjoyed the company of his friends. In all respects he was a normal man leading a normal life. All was going well, he told me, until a rival window cleaner, ignoring all the unwritten rules of the window-cleaning profession, had started to move in on his patch, causing Harry a great deal of anguish and upset and involving time and expense in defending himself. His business suffered. Harry took time off work because of stress, although he never saw a doctor.

A few years after this, his cancer was first diagnosed. It was successfully treated, and he then went on with his life for a few more years. Now it had come back and Harry knew what this meant. He had at most months to live and had reconciled himself to his situation.

"I know I'm dying, Doc, and there's nothing anyone can do about it. But I've got unfinished business before I go." It quickly became clear that he meant at the very least to threaten and perhaps even to try to kill his former rival. I didn't react straightaway, because I had never been in this situation before and wasn't quite sure what to say. While I was thinking about how to respond, sitting perched at the foot of his bed, I looked over his shoulder, and from the tenth floor of Guy's hospital tower I could see that the sun was starting to set over the city. Boats some distance below were gliding down the Thames.

I turned back to him. Perhaps he wasn't serious; perhaps this was bravado. "Are you sure about this? I mean . . ." My voice trailed off. I wasn't sure what I meant, or rather couldn't quite bring myself to put into words what it was that I wanted to say.

"Well, nothing the law can do about it, is there?" he replied.

I thought about this. In some respects he was right. He was beyond any threats of imprisonment, although looking at him, I doubted he was in a position to take anyone down, unless he had the element of surprise. He was wasting away, mostly skin and bone—but then you never knew. Perhaps all that anger would give him one last burst of strength at exactly the right moment. I asked if he knew where the man lived. He didn't, but he knew which pub he drank in. Did he have any access to weapons? He was less forthcoming on this one. A gun was the thing that I was most worried about, and who knew how easy it was to get a gun in South London?

I thought it through. My job is to act as a psychiatrist, and I had taken a psychiatric history. I had found no evidence of a mental health problem (if you discount murderous impulses toward another human as a mental health issue). And if there was no mental health problem, there was nothing for a psychiatrist to treat. And if there was nothing to treat, then my work here was done. I told Harry there was no obvious help I was able to give him, but neither could I just listen to what he had said and do nothing. I had to tell the police. He shrugged. "Do what you've got to do, Doc." So, with a sinking heart, I went back to my office and called the police.

I realized I didn't know who I was meant to ask for when I called the police. I mean, who are you meant to actually speak to? Often politicians "write to the police" when they suspect a criminal wrongdoing has been committed, but to whom do they address the letter, and where do they send it? In my case, I called the generic number for the police I found online, explained my story, and eventually spoke to a bewildered sergeant who wanted to know if a crime had actually been committed. By now this was the third time I had to tell the same story. I sighed and leaned over from my desk to switch the kettle on while the sergeant took details. I listened to the sergeant's formulaic questions, which ranged from the banal to the irrelevant, as the kettle, increasingly noisy, bubbled away.

A few days later I got a call from a senior police office on my mobile, just as I was sitting down to start clinic. I hadn't remembered giving my mobile number to anyone. The conversation was poles apart from the conversation I'd had with the confused sergeant days earlier. It reminded me of *1984,* where you eventually see the intelligent guiding hand behind Big Brother. Whatever the police had said to Harry seemed to have given him pause for thought, and he must have thought better of making threats to kill. The upshot: "Doctor, we visited your patient and gave him a talking-to. I think it fair to say he won't be attacking anyone near any pub, or anywhere else, in the near future." That was the end of that, and I heard, quite by chance when I was passing by the same ward a few weeks later, that Harry had died quietly, his family with him, without any further threats to kill anyone.

This episode stuck in my mind precisely because it is such an uncommon reaction to the realization that death is at hand. For most people, facing their own mortality is a profound, and commonly a profoundly lonely, experience. Fear of death is universal, but of the people I see who are entering their final weeks or months, fear of death is something that is not commonly expressed. I suspect this is because they are never given the opportunity to do so, and because in this country at least, we have very little culture of having these conversations. I am still haunted by a woman who I saw on my ward rounds in the general hospital some years back. She was in her sixties, with untreatable cancer and a psychiatric history of schizophrenia that had gradually alienated her from all her family and friends. She was dying alone, in a hospital ward, and her fear of her impending death was overwhelming. Every week that I saw her, ostensibly to monitor her mental health, she was more emaciated and shrunken. When I entered her room, she would be writhing in pain, although the attending medical team hadn't found a cause for her discomfort. It didn't take a psychiatrist to see that the pain was psychological, and when I tried to talk to her, she would repeat over and over again, "I'm frightened, I'm frightened."

I had little to say in reply. I understood her fear. It was hard not to be infected by it and even paralyzed by it. Although she did not want to talk much about her feelings, hers was an effective communication—at least going by my own reaction. Each time I left her room, it was with a sense of unhappiness and unease that stayed with me for hours, which no amount of eloquence could have done a better job in helping me to understand.

It was only when I eventually realized that I needed to try to stop fixing things and to de-medicalize my interactions with her that the consultations became more manageable. I would take some time to sit with her, to talk with her about her life, the things she used to enjoy doing, and at least to allow her some normal human interaction. On one occasion, I stayed to play a board game for a while, and it seemed to relax her. It wasn't medicine, not as defined these days anyway, but it achieved what no painkillers could do, which was to allow her to sit still without pain for half an hour.

More commonly, when people in their final weeks do express an anxiety, it is to wonder whether they have really lived. Bronnie Ware, an Australian nurse who looked after patients reaching the end of life, found that the number one regret of the dying was that people wished they could have lived a life truer to themselves. Sadly, most people do not, and come to regret that they allowed their true selves and their ideals to be compromised in all sorts of ways, perhaps by the company they kept or by the society they lived in. It takes great courage to live life according to your values, to put up with the sneers and ridicule (and perhaps jealousy) when your values take you outside the mainstream, and to be single-minded or principled enough to maintain those values. Very few people I know in life manage this, and I envy those who do.

End-of-life conversations are rare in hospitals. There is a squeamishness among nearly all health professionals about having the important discussions about life and death that matter to patients in their final weeks. Hospital staff feel that they have neither the skills nor the time to address the questions that patients have. Perhaps, too, it induces in the medical staff a sense of discomfort about their own mortality. Either way, the healthcare team just find it easier to focus on the technical delivery of healthcare. It is reassuring and familiar and far more controllable to focus on treatment regimens than it is to address someone's fears. Working as we do in an increasingly technocratic healthcare system, the death of a patient is seen as a failure of medical care, rather than as part of the cycle of life. Death is a topic to be avoided.

Far too few people do research in this crucial area, although one of them is the inspirational Professor Harvey Chochinov, from the University of Manitoba in Canada, whose research has been at the forefront of studying psychiatry at the end of life. When I was president of the psychiatry council at the Royal Society of Medicine, I was able to invite him over to London to speak at a conference about the end of life. For someone whose research is in an area that sounds serious and sober, he surprised me with a marvelous sense of humor. I'm not sure what I expected, but a man with a twinkle in his eye and a lively wit wasn't what I had imagined. What was also evident was a sharp intelligence and a deep compassion.

In one of his studies, Chochinov explored the desire for death among two hundred patients with a terminal illness. While over 40 percent had a fleeting wish that the end would come sooner, this feeling was persistent in only 8.5 percent of people studied. What seemed to drive a desire for death was to some extent poor family support as well as pain. Yet by far the most important factor was depression. That depression is both treatable and commonly missed in a terminally ill population is a real pity, for both the patient and their family.

Depression in the terminally ill is something health professionals rarely ask about. The common belief is that depression must be simply a normal reaction to terminal illness. Yet the prompt recognition and treatment of a mental illness can have a profound effect on someone's last days, weeks, and months as well as on the experience of their families. One of the most striking examples I remember was an elderly man on one of the oncology wards in the hospital. He had weeks to live and was being tube-fed, as he lacked the will and drive to feed himself. He was in the middle of a long ward full of patients, and since he didn't really cause anybody any trouble, instead simply sitting against the pillows and staring into his bedclothes, nobody spent much time with him. In a busy hospital environment, it's the squeaky wheel that gets the grease, and a silent, uncomplaining patient gets very little attention. The medical ward round would gather by his bedside each day, a few questions would be asked, but by then he said almost nothing, so the whole retinue of doctors, nurses, physiotherapists, pharmacists, occupational therapists, and students would sweep onto the next bed, barely delayed by their interaction with him.

By the time I saw him, it was obvious he was a dying man. It was also obvious that he was profoundly depressed, almost mute, and suffering terribly. His eyes stared ahead, with eyebrows furrowed in anguish. I think if he had been given the choice, he would have ended it all there and then, without hesitation. Instead he lay there, wasting away, his face a mask of despair. I did something then that I rarely do and decided that he needed electroconvulsive therapy (ECT). I tried to explain to him what I was proposing. He was remote, detached, indifferent. Eventually he nodded, understood, and agreed to it.

The main problem with ECT is not whether it works—in fact, for severe depression it is the most effective antidepressant there is. It is the gold standard by which all other antidepressants are measured. No, ECT has an image problem. When most people think of ECT, they think of *One Flew Over the Cuckoo's Nest*, the film starring Jack Nicholson, in which ECT is abused for the purposes of controlling unruly inmates in an asylum. This is what most people believe they know about this treatment, and the film has done more to damage the reputation of psychiatry than any single other event I can think of. It shows psychiatry as coercive and controlling, a brutal and heartless discipline. Even now, nearly fifty years after the film was made, it still gets mentioned by people who weren't alive when it was first shown in cinemas.

ECT is a strange treatment. Nobody knows how or why it works. As Andrew Scull outlines in his book *Madness in Civilization*, it was one of a number of treatments developed in the 1920s and 1930s, such as insulin comas and injections of horse serum into the spinal canal, most of them quite rightly confined to the graveyard of failed medical progress, unmourned. At the time, however, these new physical treatments for psychiatric illness were at the vanguard of scientific progress, bringing psychiatry out of the asylums and into the scientific respectability of the rest of the medical profession. First used in 1938, ECT was one such treatment and was advanced as a cure for schizophrenia. It involved passing an electrical current through the patient's brain, producing a seizure. The rationale for using ECT, long since discredited, was that schizophrenia and epilepsy could not coexist, so that by provoking a seizure, the schizophrenia would be driven out of the body. Whilst that plan met with no success, it was observed that ECT was in fact an effective treatment for depression, and thus one of medicine's most controversial treatments was born. It is used to this day, although not very commonly, saved for the most extreme and refractory cases. Nowadays, it is a very medicalized procedure, carried out under general anesthetic in a specialized ECT suite. The only evidence of a seizure is on a monitor showing the brain's electrical activity. The whole thing is over in sixty seconds, and the patient delivered back to the recovery room.

It is mainly the controversies that stop me from using this treatment more often. To start with, I am usually reluctant even to suggest using it, for fear of the patient's reaction. It must also be acknowledged that there are side effects, the most common being the effect on memory. While many doctors have argued that there is no measurable change in memory deficits, and in any case poor memory is a common symptom of the depression they are trying to treat, it cannot be denied that patients do identify memory problems. These memory deficits are not usually for facts and figures, perhaps explaining why no changes show up when memory is tested in a laboratory. Rather the deficits are usually for personally relevant memories like birthdays and wedding anniversaries, the sort of things that would never be picked up on a doctor's memory checklist. Yet still, used at the right time with the right patient, the results ECT produces are nothing short of miraculous, and on the very few times when I have used it, I have only ever had one thought: *I wish I'd done this sooner.*

So it was with my patient on the cancer ward. A typical course of treatment is a total of six to twelve applications of ECT, usually given twice weekly. Yet after the first two applications, he was sitting up in bed, smiling and talking in a hoarse whisper to the nurses, and managed a wave as I walked past him on the way to see another patient. He started to eat again and talk to other patients, and was alert and engaged. I don't think I have ever seen such an extraordinary transformation in any patient I have treated, before or since. It became a great talking point among the staff on the ward, who were astonished to see him so lively and talkative. The patient died of his disease a few weeks later, the last days of his life spent in agreeable conversation and human interaction. I shudder to think what the last days of his life would have been like if I'd done nothing. Yet I'm sure nobody would have blamed me if I'd said or done nothing at all, because "it's understandable to feel like that."

For many patients at the end of life, it is the feeling of being a nonperson that hurts the most, the impression that they may be alive but no longer count as a human being, and this thought is devastating. Here, the smallest details make the greatest difference. I believe I can do more by helping a patient reach a drink, by exchanging a pleasantry about the book they are reading or asking about the job they did, or by having a discussion about the photo of their family on the bedside table, than any of the drugs they are prescribed. These small gestures can change the patient's self-perception, and in doing so the whole mood and tone of their final days.

I remember recently sitting on the bedside of a middle-aged man, Don, as he lay in bed wearing his replica Manchester United football shirt, dying of a cancer that caused unsightly bruising all over his body, face, arms, and legs. The medical team had advised that there was no further treatment for him. His kidneys had failed, and he now needed dialysis three times per week. He had worked all his life as a driver, most recently for a delivery company. He had never married, although he had a child with a former partner, and he had now lost touch with both his ex-partner as well as his child. He lived alone in a rented housing association flat and had a few acquaintances, but no one he described as a close friend. He had no other family in England, and his dying wish was to see his brother, his only surviving relative, in Canada. Unfortunately he couldn't visit him because he was unable to afford the flight and the cost of dialysis in Canada, and his brother was too ill to travel to England. His story was hard to listen to, but it was told without self-pity. As he finished, he paused. The situation was both tragic and hopeless. I took it all in and finally said, "And you're a Manchester United fan. It doesn't get worse than that." We both laughed, and for a moment we were connected in the absurd humor and pathos of the moment, in the frailties and banalities of life. There was nothing more to do. I sat for a moment and wondered aloud whether we could apply to a charity or crowdfund a visit to Canada to see his brother one last time before he died. Although frail and exhausted, he perked up a little. He thanked me profusely, although I tried to tell him I hadn't done anything yet, but I said I would see him again after the weekend.

When I sat in the junior doctor's office on Monday afternoon going through the list of inpatients with my trainee, the patient was no longer on the board. I discovered he had died over the weekend, and I knew that this would have been on a general hospital ward, with no family or friends at his bedside. I felt a wave of melancholy at this thought, and then did what most battle-hardened doctors do, and tried not to think too hard about it. The life of a hospital doctor is punctuated with scenarios like this. I pondered the last conversation with Don and hoped that it had offered some comfort. When there is nothing more to be done medically, when we can no longer be a doctor, then it behooves us to act as fellow human beings. The ability to offer hope—realistic hope, not empty promises—is such a crucial aspect of what it is to be a good doctor. Patients need to understand that they have an ally, someone who is there for them and cares what happens to them. What you may be able to accomplish in a measurable way may be limited, but what value can you put on lessening the despair of someone's final days?

In a 1979 study from Finland published in the *American Journal of Epidemiology,* patients who received no treatment for cancer had a higher suicide rate than those given treatment. It was unclear why this was the case, since many of the suicides were within weeks of the diagnosis, when treatment may not yet have started. Perhaps these were cases where suicide took place before treatment could commence. Yet perhaps these were cases where there was a decision not to offer treatment. This could have been a practical and sensible decision, allowing better allocation of resources to other patients considered potentially treatable, not to cases considered medically hopeless. Yet individuals who feel beyond hope, considering themselves discarded by the medical profession, very quickly give up on themselves in thought, word, and deed. A more recent study in 2012 followed up on over 3.5 million people diagnosed with cancer in the United States, and showed again that the risk of suicide peaked in the first month following diagnosis, when the sense of despair and anxiety is likely to be at its highest.

The converse of course is true. I heard from Professor Chochinov about his treatment called Dignity Therapy, which is designed to address the psychological and existential distress of terminally ill patients. In this therapy, patients approaching the end of life undertake a series of interviews where they are encouraged to discuss the things in their life that matter most to them. The interviews are then transcribed and edited and can be bequeathed to family members. This is a type of personal legacy, where future generations will be able to read and understand what mattered most to the individual, and in doing so, have a better sense of who they were and what they represented in the world. For the patients themselves, approximately half reported an increased will to live, with two-thirds reporting an increased sense of purpose and meaning. It was undoubtedly helpful to their families, too, with one study showing that 78 percent of families thought that it had helped them with their grief, seeing it as a continued source of comfort for them.

I thought about Chochinov's work while I was reading about a different study in the *British Medical Journal*. This 2017 study examined the forty-eight new cancer drugs approved by the European Medicines Agency between 2009 and 2013. Depressingly, the study found that most of the drugs approved for the treatment of cancer entered the market without evidence of benefit on either survival or quality of life. In other words, despite the rapidly escalating costs for the new cancer drugs, the evidence for their benefit was very thin indeed. This appeared to be a microcosm of the practice of medicine today. Money is found for drugs that offer very little benefit at the end of life, because of the way we medicalize health, rather than give a broader consideration to patient well-being. I have no doubt that everyone who pushed for the new drugs to be released onto the market was acting with the best of intentions, trying to optimize treatment for cancer. And of course I am all for drugs that are a significant improvement on what went before, whatever the field of care. With some wishful thinking, perhaps the drugs even felt like an advance in care. Yet the evidence shows that they were not. By contrast, a form of treatment like Dignity Therapy, which can make a real difference to the experience of death, is barely thought about, let alone funded. It doesn't have the thrill of the new, of the medical breakthrough that everyone craves. That psychological therapies can have such a profound impact seems to be overlooked in the rush to endorse new medications, not out of malice or deliberate neglect but because this is what medicine has now become.

COVID

When I think back to the start of the pandemic, fragmented images come to my mind. As the storm started to gather, as we collectively held our breath, I watched a video posted on Twitter of a man in Wuhan, China, attempting to drive out of the locked-down streets. The police pull the man's car over and arrest him. There is no typical "hands up" moment, no dialogue with the would-be fugitive. Instead the man is caught in a net on the end of a pole, the sort of net that I associate with summer meadows and catching butterflies. The net is pulled over the man's head, so that the police, in full hazmat suits, can immobilize him before grappling him to the ground. This surreal sequence captures the unreal quality of what is happening. A global pandemic is sweeping through China and heading west. There is news from Hong Kong, Thailand, Korea; then suddenly it is upon us in Europe. I watch the television news as bewildered, tearful Italian doctors appear on the screen, their faces creased from wearing masks, overwhelmed by the scale of what is happening. In England and the United States, the panic is sublimated into parochial concerns about toilet paper, and for the first time in my recollection, gaps appear on super-market shelves.

Viruses are tiny particles, so small that you can't see them even under the most powerful light microscope, and they are not really alive in any normal sense of the word. They can't replicate like other living creatures. They need to enter a host cell of a real living organism, which they then hijack to produce more virus. Soon there are millions, billions of viral particles produced, waiting to be spread through the air, through blood, through touch, on into another host. Viruses have no mind, no purpose, no malevolence. We humanize the virus, call it evil, talk of fighting it, but our opponent doesn't recognize that it is trying to fight us. It is remorseless, implacable.

That a virus is bringing the world to its knees has a particular resonance. I had feared global warming, wars, terrorism perhaps, as ways in which our daily lives might change. Yet there is something about mankind's hubris being exposed by one of the tiniest particles in all of nature that is both darkly comical and desperately tragic. The virus has stripped life back to the bare essentials, and in doing so reveals our innermost characters. It does this to us as individuals and as societies, as well as in global political structures. The virus is a great revealer, as well as a great killer.

It is all action stations at the hospital. Urgent meetings are convened. The novelty of video meetings has not yet worn off. This early in the crisis, we are generous of spirit and fearful of cynicism. Many words are spoken, most of them pointless, as we avoid the obvious conclusion that nobody knows what this pandemic is going to look like. In the absence of evidence, great inferences are made. The role for psychiatry is undetermined but anticipated to be big.

Surprisingly, the first topic up for discussion is not about patients, but about how doctors and medical staff are going to cope. It is anticipated that the mental strain will prove too much. A concept is introduced that has not been used before in medicine, a term borrowed from the military, that of "moral injury." It is perhaps not surprising that a military term is used, given the language we have employed of "fighting the virus." In military terms, moral injuries are the invisible effects of conflict, the emotional effects of being required to participate in acts that go against one's moral values or witnessing such acts without preventing them. Being ethically and morally compromised, it is said, can lead to lasting shame and guilt, mental health problems, and sometimes addictions. Feelings of anger and resentment at the officers or systems that forced the individual into this situation can linger. The concern voiced in these meetings was that this was soon to be the fate of the medical staff in the hospital. They would be required to make choices about which patient got the ventilator and who would be left to die. They would not be able to look a bereaved relative in the eye and say honestly: "We did all that we could."

As the days slipped into weeks, this feared scenario was not materializing. Elsewhere in the world, many health systems were on the point of collapse and doctors were struggling to cope. In the UK, though, while intensive care doctors were busy, some overwhelmed, many of my colleagues, both in general medicine and surgery, were reporting the opposite problem, which is that they didn't have enough to do. Outpatient clinics and routine surgery and transplant lists had been canceled to create extra capacity, which it turned out we didn't need (in the first wave, at least. The second wave was altogether a more brutal and demoralizing experience). In the meanwhile, whole swaths of medical problems disappeared from healthcare settings altogether. Where were the heart attacks and strokes, asthma attacks, retinal detachments, and other urgent medical problems? They didn't seem to be coming to the hospital anymore. The number of psychiatry referrals dropped, and it seemed, at least based on my locality, that fewer patients were self-harming.

I thought back to a paper published in *The British Journal of Psychiatry* after the 9/11 attacks in the United States. The paper examined the suicide rates after the terrorist attacks and showed that suicide rates fell to their lowest level for any September in the preceding twenty-two years. This seemed to support the theories of Émile Durkheim, a French sociologist who lived in the nineteenth and early twentieth centuries. Durkheim was one of the first people to explore suicide from a sociological perspective, looking at the effects not just of the individual but of society on suicide rates. This included the effects of economics as well as other events in society. One example he highlighted was the abrupt decline in suicide rates in Europe during 1848, a year that saw a series of revolutions across the Continent. He hypothesized that in exceptional times of crisis, such as war or other conflict, people came together. While feeling alone in an atomized society presents a risk for suicide, the sense of community built up in the fight against a common enemy reduced the suicide rate. Undoubtedly the spread of Covid-19 brought on a time of crisis, and it seemed that Durkheim's theory was being proven correct. I had not forgotten the other side of his theory, though. Durkheim posited that in times of economic crisis, there is an uptick in the number of suicides. As governments across the world borrowed eye-watering amounts of money to keep the economy moving, and while economists warned of a recession bigger than anything since World War II, I worried as to whether future suicides would follow in Covid's wake.

The day before the UK government announced the lockdown, we all knew it was coming. I went to the park, a twenty-minute drive from home. I wanted to have some solitude in a wide-open space away from humanity. I was wistful, trying to absorb the fact that life was about to change, possibly for good, trying to consciously appreciate the walk. Yet the park was teeming with all the other Londoners who had had exactly the same idea. It was the first time we collectively engaged in the choreography and geometry of trying to keep two meters (a little over six feet) apart. It felt both absurd and tragic. As I walked back to the car, I noticed that nobody would pick up a Frisbee that had gone astray, for fear of becoming contaminated.

After the lockdown began the following day, the psychological effects began to appear. My wife, Sara, received a letter from an official source. It said that because of her asthma, she was in a vulnerable category were she to become infected with coronavirus, and therefore she needed to be "shielded." She needed to ensure that she did not come within two meters of any other person, including members of her immediate family, and this would need to be kept up for twelve weeks. The effect was instantaneous. Sara, a doctor herself and normally as level-headed as they come, barely saw anything beyond the word "vulnerable." I was banished to the spare room. Odd synchronized dances were carried out around the work surface in the kitchen if we found ourselves there at the same time. If I wanted to get to the fridge, Sara would scuttle around the island to the sink.

"Sara, this is absolutely nuts."

"It's government advice. I'm shielded."

"But you were sitting next to me in the car yesterday. I've not been anywhere since then."

As with many of our emotions, Sara's reaction was not based on a rational assessment of reality. This was about the feelings of powerlessness that inevitably accompany being officially labeled as vulnerable. The label introduces fear and doubt and an expectation of the worst. Over the coming weeks I spoke to many patients and friends who had similar reactions to being "shielded." There seemed to be something uniquely demoralizing about being officially categorized as vulnerable. The fear of a tap on the shoulder from the bony finger of death began to invade the thoughts of many of my patients. The coronavirus revealed the existential fear that we all carry within us.

Within the discipline of medicine itself, feelings of vulnerability abounded. Modern medicine's reputation has been built on the ability to treat infectious disease. Medicine has removed the fear of plague or of death resulting from a cut that becomes infected. Coronavirus threatened to knock the whole edifice down. The virus was behaving in strange and unpredictable ways we could barely understand, let alone control. It affected men more than women. It was particularly severe in the older population, but then suddenly, unpredictably, a fit, healthy younger person would become seriously ill. Doubt and uncertainty crept into the public psyche.

This was the worst sort of doubt. When it comes to gambling, random reinforcement is the most addictive. Random reinforcement is unpredictable intermittent winning, where the very next spin of the wheel or roll of the dice could change everything. There are no rules or ways of controlling it, which is why gamblers have superstitions, to give themselves the illusion of control. The converse is true. When a really bad outcome is possible, having little ability to predict or control it is especially demoralizing. The uncertainty itself is most destructive to people's well-being. (This reminded me of an old Jewish joke from my childhood, about a man receiving a telegram from his mother that read: *Start worrying. Details to follow.*) Coronavirus was fickle, unpredictable, with just enough uncertainty in its effects to maintain fear.

The virus seemed to introduce strange emotions in all of my colleagues. I noticed one pervasive drive was the need to feel relevant and important, to be seen as leading the charge against the virus. Medical staff posted videos and selfies of themselves in choreographed dances at work, clad in their personal protective equipment. In the real world, there was vast duplication of effort. Doctors wanted whatever new coronavirus initiative everybody else had also thought of to be their idea. I recalled the truism about psychologists, that they would rather use one another's toothbrushes than one another's rating scales. I expect it's the same everywhere. When the sands are shifting beneath our feet, we all want to feel that our lives matter.

Talking heads popped up to fill the insatiable need for Covid news. It was initially alarming, then wearying, and finally overwhelming. In an interview on the television news program *Newsnight,* Charlie Brooker, the creator of the dark futuristic drama *Black Mirror,* compared watching the news about coronavirus to eating fruit: "It's good for you up to a point, and then it gives you the shits." But we were entranced by the never-ending news, hypnotized as if by a cobra, unable to avert our gaze from the death staring at us. We all became experts in virology and epidemiology. We pinned our hopes on a vaccine. Hope is a very poor strategy for dealing with a crisis.

The effect on my patients was mixed. Some of them told me they were happier than normal, something I had not expected at the outset of the pandemic. They felt unburdened by the need for a daily commute to work and happier that they were masters of their own workplace. Control over one's working environment plays an undervalued but very important role in our health and well-being. In the well-known White-hall study, a group of researchers examined the incidence of heart disease in civil servants working at Whitehall, the heart of the UK government. The researchers found that the extent to which you could control your work environment—in other words, when and how you did your work—correlated with future risk of heart disease. Employees who had little control over their work were more stressed than those who had more. This lack of control over the work predicted a higher rate of coronary artery disease in the follow-up period. So it was for some of my patients, for the first time tasting a greater degree of autonomy, feeling more trusted, more in control, and more fulfilled.

Even more surprising were some of my patients with anxiety disorders and depression, who told me that they were tolerating the lockdown well; some of them were even enjoying it. Everyone was now living in their world. Nobody was going out more than they were or having a better time. For once, these patients were part of the greater experience of humanity, not the forgotten and marginalized minority. A couple of patients said they had been dreading a catastrophe like this for so long that now that it had arrived, it was almost a relief. Their focus was no longer on the worrying and uncertainty, but rather on trying to make the best of it.

Most commonly, though, patients were starting to suffer. I called up one of my outpatients, whom I had first seen a few months previously. He had been referred with persistent low mood and anxiety, but also had unexplained itchiness. At first, the medical team wondered if the itchiness was a symptom of liver or kidney disease, but all the investigations drew a blank, and it remained unexplained. He was in his mid-twenties, thin, somewhat ill at ease sitting on the chair opposite my desk. I expect he realized that drug use was the cause of all his problems, because it didn't take me long to work it out, but he had allowed himself to be put through a round of investigations rather than face the shame of telling his doctors. Perhaps there was an element of wishful thinking or denial, too. But once we got talking about the drug use, once it was out in the open, it was obviously a relief for him to be able to tell me. He used drugs most days because he was bored; he was using to fill a void in his life. He had no family to whom he was close, no real friends to speak of, and no social life. He lived alone with his dog, and although he had a clerical job to occupy him in the day, he had nothing to do in the evenings, which is when he would start using. We developed a treatment plan based on increasing his social contact and structuring his life so that he didn't need to rely on drugs to get him through the long evenings alone. He told me that the plan had been working well until the lockdown and the enforced isolation. Boredom became his companion once more, and before long he was using drugs again. I had little doubt he was understating the extent to which he was taking drugs. Perhaps he didn't want to disappoint me. More likely he didn't want to admit it to himself. Either way, it's never easy to watch a patient regress.

Others of my patients became more paranoid. Isolation brings out such traits in people. I recall one of my elderly relatives becoming more paranoid in her old age. Even when she was younger, she was a bit mistrustful. She was always sure the cleaner was stealing from her or the grocer was putting lower quality produce in her shopping bag. When she was older and widowed, she would telephone to inform us that someone had entered her apartment during the night and taken some soap or moved her shoes. We all assumed she was becoming demented and the paranoia was just one sign of it, but once she moved to a residential home, to our surprise the paranoia disappeared. Having another form of human contact is helpful in what you might call a quick sanity check. It allows for triangulation of our thoughts or emotions, to ensure we haven't quietly slipped our moorings. We have all had the experience of ruminating over a comment that someone has made, turning it this way and that, and eventually imbuing it with a meaning that it never had. We need someone reliable to tell us when we are overreacting. Isolation can remove these checks and balances, revealing a default way of thinking that leads to mistrust and hostility.

Others of my patients started to get more withdrawn and depressed. The lack of social contact was difficult, but being put out of work or furloughed (the latter a word that most of us had never heard of prior to Covid-19, and which to me sounded vaguely equine) was particularly demoralizing for some. Time gaped, and into that time bled all the doubt and uncertainty that hitherto had been kept at bay by the distractions of everyday life. For those predisposed to anxiety, the advent of Covid-19 led to anxious thoughts about when and how it would all end.

For those prone to depression, it induced feelings of helplessness, entrapment, and despair.

In government, coronavirus revealed and amplified the shortcomings of politicians, presidents, and whole political systems. It was disconcerting for politicians to face a crisis over which they had such limited control, and where the adverse outcomes of any decisions were measurable in daily excess deaths. Some politicians tried to obfuscate and deny the truth, even though they surely must have known that the truth would out. Others believed that by force of will they could wish the problem away, only to discover that wishful thinking is an even worse strategy than hope. The more authoritarian the politicians' instincts, the more they tried to face down the virus rather than actually engaging with the science, the worse the problems seemed to get. Lying in bed one night, I wondered what was passing through the minds of world leaders as they lay in bed. Did they feel fear or guilt, indifference or fatalism, panic, or a calm born of moral rectitude? I did not envy them. I expect they tried not to think about the human cost of their decisions at all.

And for me? I worried about my parents in Manchester, whom I hadn't seen in months. I found something claustrophobic in only ever being at my home or place of work, with no friends, football matches, cafés, pubs, or holidays. There was a continual sense of time passing. The sun rose and the sun set. Days passed. I could hear the birds singing in the trees. Each night as I lay in bed, I would wonder whether my life had had value that day. These ruminations were sometimes accompanied by a jolt of anxiety, a deep unease. This was coronavirus as the great revealer. I realized that I struggle in my own company, I fear loneliness, I fear unproductive old age, I fear dying.

I feared, too, for humanity. But I believe that we are a proud and resilient species. Perhaps coronavirus will be an opportunity to rethink our interactions with one another, make us into a more connected, generous, and giving society. For all our human foibles, we want to have a sense of belonging, to be able to contribute to the greater good, and one day to look back at our lives and be able to say that the world was a better place for our passage through it. Maybe the coming years will bring that change. Perhaps coronavirus will lead us to a more just, more interconnected, more equal society. Maybe together we will be up to the challenges of global warming, poverty, and inequality.

Coronavirus, the revealer and agent of change. For a time it stripped us bare. We fell back to the essence of the lives we have built for ourselves. It has made me understand more about myself. I realize that I fundamentally like people. I identify with many of the problems that I see in my clinics, even if I have never experienced them. I feel a great sympathy for humanity, for our fears and vulnerabilities, our insecurities, the sadness of our predicament, the essential humanness of my fellow travelers on this planet. Perhaps that's why I'm a psychiatrist. I want to try to help them.

EPILOGUE

Psychiatrists don't often get thank-you letters. For most people, a visit to a psychiatrist is something they'd rather put behind them, so when I saw a letter waiting for me in my pigeonhole, in a hand-addressed cream envelope, I couldn't even guess what it was about. With some effort, I ripped through the envelope, narrowly avoiding tearing the letter inside. The letter was from a patient I'd long since forgotten. I'd met her only once, and that was four years earlier, so I looked up her notes to remind myself why I'd seen her. She was a nurse who had come to see me with a history of depression. Although she had been given antidepressants regularly over the years, she wasn't sure they had helped much, and her depression seemed to come and go of its own accord. She was worried that she had a treatment-resistant depression, and this fear had come to dominate her life.

After a consultation with her, I came to the conclusion that the reasons antidepressants hadn't worked was that she hadn't been depressed in the first place. She may well have had an episode of depression some years previously, which had responded to treatment, but every passing emotion since then seemed to end with her getting medicated. People commonly forget after they've been depressed that it's normal to cry when you're heartbroken and feel sad when things aren't going your way. It's tempting to attribute those feelings to relapsing depression, and doctors often end up agreeing. Diagnoses like depression are not just labels—they are sticky labels, hard to get rid of. They can end up doing a lot of harm by convincing people they are unwell and ultimately helpless in the face of life's problems. My advice to her was to get on with her life, to live it and enjoy it. After all, she was healthy and didn't really have problems except for the ones she herself was generating. I wished her well and discharged her from my clinic after one visit.

She wrote to say that she had found my summary of our appointment in the back of a filing cabinet while she was searching for some mortgage documents. She wanted to tell me that after that appointment, she had thought more about what I had said. She realized that she had overcomplicated her life by a preoccupation with mental illness. With a different perspective, she could see that she was fundamentally well—at worst prone to self-limiting problems. Employing this new way of thinking, she saw little reason not to accept her boyfriend's marriage proposal. She had now been married for three years and had since had twins. Life was going well for her, and she thought I might like to know.

I was delighted to read the letter. It seemed strange to think that a long-forgotten appointment, with a patient whose name I couldn't even remember, had made such an impression on her, and had even led to marriage and children. On the one hand, I hadn't really done anything. I hadn't made a clever diagnosis or used a special new imaging technique. I hadn't treated her with the latest and most expensive medication. If I had, I bet the improvement in her condition would have been considered great medicine. What I had done, though, was take a careful history of her problems, make an attempt to understand her life's experiences, and come to the conclusion that she had the opposite of a health problem. Others previously had taken a different view, had assessed only a snapshot of her symptoms, and had prescribed different courses of antidepressants.

It brought to mind something I read when I was a medical student, in a dusty old book that I found in the library while I was preparing for my final exams. It concerned a debate that was said to have taken place at the British Medical Association in the late 1940s, concerning whether medicine was a science or an art. I remember reading and then rereading the paragraph. The question made no sense to me. I simply didn't understand how it could have been asked. I was knee-deep in textbooks on pathology, biochemistry, physiology, anatomy, and surgery. I was learning to read X-rays and hearing about a technique new at the time, MRI, with its beautiful images and ability to peer directly into the body itself. Medicine was so obviously a science that I struggled to understand how intelligent people thought this question worthy of a debate. I read on, flipping the page to see that in this debate, by a very narrow margin, medicine had been declared a science. *Good,* I thought, but still, nearly half the audience thought that it wasn't. I shook my head and assumed the debate was conducted among doctors from a lost generation. Doctors in strange frock coats with their superstitious ways, with their purges and poultices and leeches, which had nothing to do with medicine as I was learning it now.

Over time, though, I have come to realize that while the underpinning of medicine is a science, the practice of medicine is an art. I am very respectful of the science, of course. I marvel at the innovations in healthcare. I read avidly about genomics, targeted monoclonal antibodies, surgical advances. Yet the people who benefit from these advances are only a small proportion of people presenting with illness to their doctor. Unfortunately medicine has sold itself on the notion that this is real medicine. There are ecstatic documentaries following the heroics of surgical teams, featuring images of spirals of DNA. It is unsurprising, given that this is what the public have been exposed to, that this is what they think medicine is. There is a belief that medicine is based largely on pipettes and test tubes, biopsies and pathology slides, imaging and pinpoint surgery, a belief so pervasive that it has largely gone unchallenged.

I remember as a medical student being sent to a hospital that was miles out of London for my pediatric training. The life of a medical student is often quite dull and entails a persistent feeling of uselessness—a sense that one is getting under everyone's feet and not really contributing to the patient's welfare. I was made to turn up to endless clinics and sit quietly observing. It was not an inspirational or even an effective way to learn. Boredom was a fairly constant companion. Some of the better doctors would send you off to speak to the patient or parents alone; some would remember you were there from time to time and engage in a cursory discussion of the patient after he or she had left; and some would ignore you entirely, treating you like a piece of furniture. I was in one of the latter type of clinics, waiting for it to end or to be told to go for lunch. I wriggled on the chair, aware that my backside was numb. A number of children with asthma were being seen one after another in the clinic. When the session was finally over, I asked the registrar running it if he enjoyed his job, and whether he would recommend pediatrics as a career. It was as if the dam had been breached. He told me how he had bitterly regretted his career choice. He believed it would be about his saving lives, about grateful parents, the drama and excitement of pressured decisions. Instead, his life was about liaising with schools, meetings with social services, and reassuring anxious parents, and he hated every minute of it. Nobody had told him that this was medicine. He had realized far too late that medicine is not the heroics, the flash of insight and genius that saves the day. That makes good television but represents only a tiny minority of our encounters with patients.

Healthcare has become ever more specialized, ever more fragmented into specialist teams. Knowledge among specialists is getting deeper and narrower, but at the cost of losing the broader picture. Many times I have been asked to see patients passed along by five or six different specialists before being sent to me. Each appointment has cost the patient time and emotional energy, and yet when I read the specialists' reports, they nearly all say the same thing. They can state with certainty what the patient's problem is *not,* which is anything to do with the organ they specialize in. Sometimes they reach this conclusion only after investigating and treating spurious findings on scans or in blood tests. They suggest another specialist to look elsewhere for the cause of the patient's troubles. Everyone is secure in their own circumscribed specialist area, and increasingly helpless outside of it.

Medicine is practiced on the assumption that when a patient presents with symptoms, it is because of an underlying disease. The messy narrative, the imprecision of the patient's perception of what is wrong with them—all this must yield to the probing clarity of the doctor. Doctors want to cut through the noise, to find the signal. One study showed that when a patient first sits down for an appointment, a doctor will typically interrupt after eleven seconds. The doctor is setting the agenda, not the patient. The doctor's agenda is to work out where the pathology is, a laser-like search to force the body to give up its secrets, through a combination of close questioning and targeted investigations. It is an attempt to make order out of chaos. The fog lifts and a diagnosis appears, its focus sharpening in the sunlight.

The problem with this approach is that the real world is swimming in shades of gray. Patients present with symptoms that have nothing to do with disease or diagnosis. Understanding the patient's agenda allows for a far more productive consultation. It allows you to address directly what patients are worried that their problem might be, and often this is not something that the doctor could ever guess. I recall seeing a young woman with headaches, which did not much concern the doctor who was seeing her, but she eventually persuaded him to do brain scans and various other investigations. Despite the care she had received, she felt "dismissed" by the doctor, something I felt was a little unfair given that he had investigated her quite thoroughly. Yet she said that he did so grudgingly, perfunctorily. Finally, when the results came back as normal, she heard him say, "It's all good news. There's nothing wrong with you."

Yet she did think something was wrong with her, because she still had the headaches. As we talked, I asked if she didn't trust the doctor who had investigated her. She told me it wasn't that. "Well," I said, "you've obviously thought about this a great deal. What's your theory about the headaches?" She was a little embarrassed to say, knowing it to be an overreaction but feeling a genuine fear. She told me about a university friend who had to drop out last term because of a brain tumor. She didn't know what had happened to him—they weren't especially close—but the episode had left her in a high state of anxiety. She simply needed reassuring that she didn't have a brain tumor. When she was provided that reassurance, her headache simply melted away.

Doctors often have very little time to *really* talk to patients. There are huge pressures on throughput in outpatient clinics, an insatiable demand that is almost impossible to meet. This demonstrates the truism of "more haste, less speed," because it is not cost effective. We already know about the extra billions spent every year on unnecessary investigations. We have seen the costs of psychiatric problems complicating long-term disease, both health costs and financial. We see the costs in end-of-life care, in our failure to understand why patients make the decisions that they do and fail to take their prescribed medications.

If you've had a row with someone about changing their mind, you will know that the starting point is to listen and understand their position. Changing people's minds is based on someone's having felt heard, rather than having been shouted down. Only once they feel you have listened to them will they prepare to listen to you. So it is in medicine. If you want to treat a patient effectively, particularly if you want a patient to understand your point of view, you need to be listening more than talking. Yet we know that doctors spend a considerable amount of time in a consultation doing the talking, interrupting patients early and often.

Most doctors know all this already. But knowing it and practicing it are two different things. Despite what we know about illness and patient behavior, the practice of medicine is consistently skewed toward a rationalistic, scientific perspective. This is more pronounced in secondary care, where doctors are more likely to believe that their role is to deal with diseased bodies, not troubled minds. It is an understandable attempt to gain control of the problem, in which life's cares are reducible to a diagnosis (and later to a diagnostic billing code). This approach may help the doctors but fundamentally does not serve the patients, because a simplistic understanding of a patient's problems will lead to a simplistic solution. Effective medicine is about understanding the context of someone's life. It's about patients feeling understood. An inability to get this is the commonest reason for someone using alternative or complementary medicine. Patients may respect the technical ability of medicine but not its human heart.

Because I work in a teaching hospital, I am allocated medical students. I enjoy the experience, because medical students have not usually had their common sense educated out of them yet and often ask searching questions. Yet the drive for clarity and simplicity is strong. Teaching medical students about treatments for medical conditions is usually to elicit single-word answers, commonly in the form of drug names. I try to explain, for example, that the treatment for depression is not simply antidepressants, or at least not these drugs by themselves, but is rather an understanding of the individual's lifestyle, support, employment, and drug use—all manner of things that may need to be optimized to effect a recovery. The same is true for physical health problems. The solution to treating pain is not painkillers alone, but understanding the context of the pain, any associated emotional triggers: whether the patient feels they have any control over the pain, what they think the pain means, and what their fears of it are. Medicine that is practiced without a wider appreciation of the context of the symptoms or the psychological aspects of them is literally mindless. Decades of scientific reductionism of medicine has brought us to this point.

Doctors, when they are sure they are not being overheard, will talk of "heart-sink patients." These are patients who make a doctor's heart sink as they enter the clinic room. Previously these patients had bulging medical folders, and nowadays associated with them are megabytes of electronic notes that take an age to load. They keep returning to the doctor with ongoing symptoms, which the doctor is unable to resolve, and which medical specialists keep sending back to the GP without a diagnosis. A bit of back pain, headaches that won't seem to go away, dizziness, sinus trouble, pelvic pain, exhaustion, the sensation of a lump in the throat, a chronic cough, persistent itchiness. Among the medical profession, such patients induce a sense of helplessness and frustration, because there are few things that doctors dislike more than a patient who won't get better. That the patient keeps coming back is something of a provocation, a reminder of the doctor's impotence. It represents the failure of current ways of practicing medicine to address the problems with which many patients present. The patients are thought of as "not really ill," despite their going to their doctor for help with symptoms. It's clear that something about the way we think about and practice medicine has gone wrong.

A urologist friend and colleague of mine, Jonathan Glass, told me about his thoughts (later published in his excellent blog) about the heart-sink patient. One week, the heart-sink patient was the theme for the weekly urology meeting that his department have held for years. Members of his department took turns presenting their difficult patients. Jonathan decided to turn things on their head by seeing things from a patient's point of view. He coined the term "heart-sink doctor." These are the doctors who make patients groan as soon as they enter the consulting room. Patients realize straightaway that the consultation will be perfunctory and the doctor will invest little emotional energy or even basic interest in them. Heart-sink doctors "make no attempt to discover anything more about the person in front of them other than their presenting symptoms . . . they are protocol driven and fail to individualise the care they offer. They are looking to refer the patient on to another specialty at the earliest opportunity."

It is the ability to find out about the patient in front of you, with genuine interest and curiosity, that is difficult to teach and yet without which one can't be an effective clinician. Without understanding the patient's life, one can't understand the meaning of a symptom and why that patient might fear it. Normal twitching of the eyelids carries a very different meaning to someone whose relative has had multiple sclerosis than to someone who hasn't slept properly in a few nights. Without knowing their values and world view, one cannot understand why individuals might not want to take the prescribed medication or have the treatment that a doctor think that they must have. What doctors see as noncompliance with treatment is usually a point of view that the doctor has not yet understood.

I have met very few bad doctors in my career. Nearly all the doctors I have met have been principled, driven, and hardworking, motivated by a desire to improve the lives of the people they care for. It is just that the system we have created for ourselves, the system we call medicine, has drifted off course. The former Israeli ambassador to the United States and the United Nations, Abba Eban, once said that "a consensus means that everyone agrees to say collectively what no one believes individually." The consensus in medicine, believed by almost nobody individually, but practiced almost universally, is that more medicine is better medicine, the fallacy that more investigations and more treatment lead to improved outcomes. A campaign called Choosing Wisely in North America has tried to address this over recent years, spreading throughout many Western countries, yet the pull to overinvestigate and overprescribe remains strong.

I have spent many years of my career picking up the pieces from the consequences of this type of approach. I think of Gavin, a forty-four-year-old with persistent migraines. He told me that they first began suddenly one morning ten years earlier and had persisted ever since. They stopped him from working, had nearly ruined his relationship with his wife, and had caused his friends to drift away. He recalled that fateful morning when they started, without warning, as he woke up. He told me that he must have been grinding his jaw during the night, because it ached as he woke up, and his head was pounding. He began to recount his story.

Gavin was a meek and sensitive man. He gave the impression of someone kind yet timid, struggling to balance his priorities in life—his work, partner, and family—without causing offense to any of them. Against his wife's wishes, he had been looking after his mother in her final illness. His wife was not supportive. She couldn't see why other family members wouldn't help, why it was always his job. She told him that he had responsibilities to her. But even as he looked after his ailing mother, his brother became convinced this was Gavin's attempt to take all of the inheritance that would be shortly due. His brother was mistrustful to such a degree that there began months of family infighting.

When their mother died and the will was read, somehow Gavin

ended up with nothing. There was no explanation. He just couldn't make sense of it. He speculated that maybe his mother thought his brother's financial need was greater, or perhaps (and he thought this far more likely) his brother had hectored and cajoled their mother until she simply gave in and agreed to change her will. Gavin found it all but impossible to express his upset. He told me that he had dreams in which he shouted at his brother, saying all the things he could never say to him in real life. He ground his jaw at night. He became tense, edgy, and filled with foreboding throughout the day. His relationship with his brother fractured and eventually they stopped talking ("He's dead to me now").

Gavin saw his doctor and was referred to neurology in his local hospital for investigation of his headaches. He received an MRI of his head and an extensive range of blood tests. When all these investigations came back as normal, he was given Botox injections, medications, and a TENS machine to try to control the pain. A TENS machine is a little box that delivers mild electric shocks via pads on the skin to try to block the pain signals traveling to the brain. It is based on the gate theory of pain, where light touch preferentially gets passed up to the brain and closes the gate to pain sensations.

Nothing worked. All along, he had been trying to tell the doctors his theory, that his headaches could have been the result of his argument with his brother and being cut out of his mother's will. Yet the idea was not even discussed. It was simply ignored altogether. It took ten years and a change of hospital and medical team before anyone asked about his own thoughts about his illness. Finally, many years down the line, with his life now defined by his inability to do almost anything, he was getting the help that he had tried to ask for all along. "Ten years of my life," he said, balling up an imaginary piece of paper and tossing it into the bin in the corner of the room. "All those wasted appointments, all those investigations and treatments."

I thought about Gavin after the appointment. It was the visual representation that stuck in my mind. The balled-up piece of paper that represented the years of his life, tossed away. It was difficult to explain how this could happen except to say that the practice of medicine discourages complex psychological explanations of health problems in favor of simplistic medical ones.

It is apparent that our way of practicing medicine perpetuates a system of healthcare that does not fit the majority of patients who come to see us. Over the twenty years I have worked as a psychiatrist, I have come to understand the wisdom of the physicians who preceded me, who have always understood that medicine is first and foremost about people. Every generation needs to relearn this. Each generation believes that its technological sophistication renders human interaction secondary in the process of diagnosis and treatment.

Far from being peripheral to medicine, psychiatry *is* medicine. And yet psychiatry is done superficially, if at all, in most acute hospitals in the country. In the UK we spend £8 to £13 billion extra per annum because of our failure to address the mental health needs of people with long-term physical health conditions. This includes £3 billion annually in needless investigations of people presenting to doctors with physical conditions, but for whom the cause is psychological, such as in Gavin's case. In the United States, it is estimated that the costs of medically unexplained symptoms are $256 billion per annum. At every stage of the patient pathway, from visits to primary care, emergency care, outpatient visits, and hospital admissions, people with medically unexplained symptoms have more visits and higher costs.

I have spent a career observing the truth of the statistics—that people with depression die sooner of their medical problems than people without depression; that people presenting with symptoms to their GP commonly do not have any physical explanation to account for them. I have come to understand how our mental health and personalities dictate not only our experience of symptoms but also the outcomes of our physical health problems, throughout the whole of the lifespan.

It is true that we are the prisoners and products of our personalities and minds, in our physical health as much as in life generally, although this need not be so. My experience has been that in helping people to break out of those prisons, in understanding the ways in which the body and the mind interact, the art and science of medicine can be combined to become far more powerful and effective than either alone.

ACKNOWLEDGMENTS

When I decided to write a book, to develop my ideas about how our physical health is inextricably linked with our mental health, I thought the process would be simple. I imagined that I would write a book and then choose which publisher would print it. Naïvety like that can sometimes be an advantage in life; otherwise it would be hard to get anything started. But there comes a point, fairly quickly in my case, when the realities of writing a book and the arcane processes of publishing become apparent. Here it was my great good fortune to have met my agent Jonathan Conway, one of the kindest, gentlest, and wisest people I know, to help give shape and focus to the book, and to believe in my writing when it was at its most raw. It has also been a privilege to have worked with my wonderful editors, Caroline Sutton at Avery and Mike Harpley at Atlantic. The book has benefited in countless ways from their insights and probing questions, their eye for detail, and their belief in the book. I would also like to acknowledge the work of my agent in the United States, George Lucas, and an assistant editor at Avery, Hannah Steigmeyer, for their kindness and efficiency, both with a tendency to reply to emails almost before I have sent them.

Several of my colleagues around the country have been so generous with their time in discussing and helping me to develop ideas. Professor Michael Sharpe in Oxford; Professor Alan Carson in Edinburgh; Dr.

Annabel Price in Cambridge in pyschiatry; Miss Clare Adams, surgeon in Harrogate; and Dr. Gideon Paul, cardiologist in Israel, all spent time talking to me about concepts in the book, for nothing more than the love of medicine. Closer to home in London, many others made a number of helpful contributions: Mr. Jonathan Glass, a urologist (but in my mind practically a psychiatrist himself); Professor Alex Leff, Professor Ros Ferner, Dr. Guy Leschziner, and Dr. Paul Bentley in neurology; Dr. David Game and Dr. Rishi Pruthi in nephrology; Professor Luigi Gnudi in diabetes and metabolic medicine; Dr. Siobhan Gee, pharmacist; Dr. Renata Pires, Dr. Daniela Alves, and Dr. Dorota Jagielska-Hall in psychology; Dr. Tim Segal in neuropsychiatry; and Professor Trudie Chalder in the persistent physical symptoms unit. I would like to acknowledge the patients I have seen over the years, for whom it has been a privilege to try to offer some help to in difficult times. I am also grateful to my hospital, the South London and Maudsley NHS Foundation Trust, who have been exemplary employers, and Guy's and St. Thomas' NHS Foundation Trust, where I spend much of my working week.

There is a moment while writing a book when the chapters must leave the safety of one's computer, to meet the harsh glare of public criticism. It is always an unsettling moment, and for this reason I am eternally grateful to my sister, Kate Fulton, my biggest cheerleader, who was the first to read and critique any chapter, and did so in a way that encouraged rather than demoralized me. I am also grateful to my friend Dan Green, whose passion for books made him the obvious choice for another opinion, which he gave with clarity and humor.

I would like to end with some final acknowledgments, some distant and some close. As to the distant ones, much of this book was written on my daily commutes to and from work, on the London Underground Northern Line. Wedged into a seat or standing up and trying to type one-handed holding my iPad in the other hand, I was always coy about passengers reading over my shoulder, even though the book was intended for the public to read. But to my fellow travelers and sufferers of the Northern Line, you can buy your own copy now.

Finally to my family. My parents have been endlessly supportive, never slow to tell me what they think of my ideas but proud to see it all come together. To my in-laws, for everything they have done over the years. To my sister, Kate, and brother, Tim, who I count among my closest friends. To my four boys, who make everything worthwhile, and who like to point out my grammatical errors as they walk past the computer, particularly my excessive use of commas. And to my wife, Sara, my North Star and love of my life, hematologist, accomplisher of tasks, and my inspiration.

NOTES

JOURNEY

6 **little evidence that such analysis improves our long-term health:** Eric A. Finkelstein et al., "Effectiveness of Activity Trackers with and without Incentives to Increase Physical Activity (TRIPPA): A Randomised Controlled Trial." *The Lancet: Diabetes and Endocrinology* 4, no. 12 (2016): P983–95; doi:10.1016/S2213 -8587(16)30284-4.

6 **people were sicker and more disabled than their forebears:** Lois M. Verbrugge, "Longer Life but Worsening Health? Trends in Health and Mortality of Middle-Aged and Older Persons." *The Milbank Memorial Fund Quarterly. Health and Society* 62, no. 3 (1984): 475–519; doi:10.2307/3349861.

6 **the number of people permanently limited by disability increased by 37 percent:** A. Colvez and M. Blanchet, "Disability Trends in the United States Population 1966–76: Analysis of Reported Causes." *American Journal of Public Health* 71, no. 5 (1981): 464–71; doi:10.2105/ajph.71.5.464.

7 **low back pain is estimated to cost the healthcare system over $100 billion per year:** Jeffrey N. Katz, "Lumbar Disc Disorders and Low-Back Pain: Socioeconomic Factors and Consequences." *Journal of Bone and Joint Surgery* 88, suppl. 2 (2006): 21–24; doi:10.2106/JBJS.E.01273.

7 **Studies in Western countries:** Keith T. Palmer et al., "Back Pain in Britain: Comparison of Two Prevalence Surveys at an Interval of 10 Years." *BMJ* 320, no. 7249 (2000): 1577–78; doi:10.1136/bmj.320.7249.1577; Janet K. Freburger et al., "The Rising Prevalence of Chronic Low Back Pain." *Archives of Internal Medicine* 169, no. 3 (2009): 251–58; doi:10.1001/archinternmed.2008.543.

7 **little doubt that beliefs and attitudes toward back pain:** Heiner Raspe, Angelika Hueppe, and Hannelore Neuhauser, "Back Pain, a Communicable Disease?" *International Journal of Epidemiology* 37, no. 1 (2008): 69–74; doi:10.1093/ije /dym220.

9 **people who were recovering from a heart attack:** K. J. Petrie et al., "Role of Patients' View of Their Illness in Predicting Return to Work and Functioning after Myocardial Infarction: Longitudinal Study." *BMJ* 312, no. 7040 (1996): 1191–94; doi:10.1136/bmj.312.7040.1191.

9 **Physical activity after a heart attack:** Örjan Ekblom et al., "Increased Physical Activity Post–Myocardial Infarction Is Related to Reduced Mortality: Results from the SWEDEHEART Registry." *Journal of the American Heart Association* 7, no. 24 (2018): e010108; doi:10.1161/JAHA.118:010108.

STIGMA

17 **particularly people who are socially isolated and lonely, are at higher risk of suicide:** Raffaella Calati et al., "Suicidal Thoughts and Behaviors and Social Isolation: A Narrative Review of the Literature." *Journal of Affective Disorders* 245 (2019): 653–67; doi:10.1016/j.jad.2018:11.022.

CULTURE

27 **illness was the consequences of a brain disorder:** Sandra D. Haynes and T. L. Bennett, "Historical Perspective and Overview," in Thomas L. Bennett, ed., *The Neuropsychology of Epilepsy* (Springer, 1992): 3–15.

28 **Rick J. Carlson said in his 1975 book:** Rick J. Carlson, *The End of Medicine* (Wiley, 1975): 202.

33 **an underlying physical cause was shown in only 16 percent of the cases:** K. Kroenke and A. D. Mangelsdorff, "Common Symptoms in Ambulatory Care: Incidence, Evaluation, Therapy, and Outcome." *American Journal of Medicine* 86, no. 3 (1989): 262–66; doi:10.1016/0002-9343(89)90293-3.

33 **A study carried out in London:** C. Nimnuan, M. Hotopf, and S. Wessely, "Medically Unexplained Symptoms: An Epidemiological Study in Seven Specialities." *Journal of Psychosomatic Research* 51, no. 1 (2001): 361–67; doi:10.1016/s0022-3999(01)00223-9.

34 **just 48 percent of outpatient attendees:** A. M. van Hemert et al., "Psychiatric Disorders in Relation to Medical Illness Among Patients of a General Medical Outpatient Clinic." *Psychological Medicine* 23, no. 1 (1993): 167–73; doi:10.1017/s0033291700038952.

34 **in the UK are estimated to cost over £3 billion per year:** Chris Naylor et al., "Bringing Together Physical and Mental Health: A New Frontier for Integrated Care," King's Fund, March 2016; https://www.kingsfund.org.uk/sites/default/files/field/field_publication_file/Bringing-together-Kings-Fund-March-2016_1.pdf.

34 **scanning patients with daily headaches would be reassuring for sufferers:** Louise Howard et al., "Are Investigations Anxiolytic or Anxiogenic? A Randomised Controlled Trial of Neuroimaging to Provide Reassurance in Chronic Daily

Headache." *Journal of Neurology, Neurosurgery, and Psychiatry* 76, no. 11 (2005): 1558–64; doi:10.1136/jnnp.2004.057851.

34 draws a distinction between illness and disease: Michael Sharpe and Monica Greco, "Chronic Fatigue Syndrome and an Illness-Focused Approach to Care: Controversy, Morality and Paradox." *Medical Humanities* 45, no. 2 (2019): 183–87; doi:10.1136/medhum-2018-011598.

38 Guy's physicians are famous throughout the medical world: Riaz Agha and Maliha Agha, "A History of Guy's, King's and St. Thomas' Hospitals from 1649 to 2009: 360 Years of Innovation in Science and Surgery." *International Journal of Surgery* 9, no. 5 (2011): 414–27; doi:10.1016/j.ijsu.2011.04.002.

38 Astley Cooper: Rikki Singal et al., "Sir Astley Paston Cooper: History, English Surgeon and Anatomist." *Indian Journal of Surgery* 73, no. 1 (2011): 82–84; doi:10.1007/s12262-010-0177-2.

MELANCHOLIA

47 Andrew Scull points out in his book: Andrew Scull, *Hysteria: The Biography* (Oxford University Press, 2009).

50 an animal model for human depression: M. E. P. Seligman, "Learned Helplessness." *Annual Review of Medicine* 23, no. 1 (1972): 407–12; doi:10.1146/annurev .me.23.020172.002203.

ALTRUISM

57 approximately 5,000 people currently waiting: NHS Blood and Transplant, "Organ Donation and Transplantation Activity Report 2019/20," 2020; https://nhs btdbe.blob.core.windows.net/umbraco-assets-corp/19220/activity-report -2019-2020.pdf.

57 the average wait time for a kidney to become available is in the order of four years: A. J. Matas et al., "OPTN/SRTR 2012 Annual Data Report: Kidney." *American Journal of Transplantation* 14, suppl. 1 (2014): 11–44; doi:10.1111/ajt.12579.

61 "call to self-sacrifice": N. Scheper-Hughes, "The Tyranny of the Gift: Sacrificial Violence in Living Donor Transplants." *American Journal of Transplantation* 7, no. 3 (2007): 507–11; doi:10.1111/j.1600-6143.2006.01679.x.

62 *Thinking, Fast and Slow*: Daniel Kahneman, *Thinking, Fast and Slow* (Macmillan, 2011).

63 in a 1994 paper by Veronica Denes-Raj and Seymour Epstein: V. Denes-Raj and S. Epstein, "Conflict Between Intuitive and Rational Processing: When People Behave Against Their Better Judgment." *Journal of Personality and Social Psychology* 66, no. 5 (1994): 819–29; doi:10.1037//0022-3514.66.5.819.

66 colleagues of mine at Guy's Hospital: Najma H. Maple et al., "Understanding Risk in Living Donor Nephrectomy." *Journal of Medical Ethics* 36, no. 3 (2010): 142–47; doi:10.1136/jme.2009.031740.

74 money will resolve all our cares and lead to happiness is a fallacy: P. Brickman, D. Coates, and R. Janoff-Bulman, "Lottery Winners and Accident Victims: Is Happiness Relative?" *Journal of Personality and Social Psychology* 36, no. 8 (1978): 917–27; doi:10.1037//0022-3514.36.8.917.

SUICIDE

90 In the United States, it is estimated that up to 47 percent of adults are lonely: John Murphy, "New Epidemic Affects Nearly Half of American Adults," MDLinx, January 10, 2019; https://www.mdlinx.com/internal-medicine/article /3272.

91 One study reported that over 9 million adults in the UK are often or always lonely: British Red Cross, "Trapped in a Bubble: An Investigation into Triggers for Loneliness in the UK," December 2016; https://www.redcross.org.uk/-/media /documents/about-us/research-publications/health-and-social-care/co-op-trapped -in-a-bubble-report.pdf?la=en&hash=5EFA679100B4EBCF0FEB705EB582E277 5BD83844.

91 television or pets are the main form of company: Age UK, "Evidence Review: Loneliness in Later Life," updated July 2015; https://www.ageuk.org.uk/globalas sets/age-uk/documents/reports-and-publications/reports-and-briefings/health -wellbeing/rb_june15_lonelines_in_later_life_evidence_review.pdf.

91 chronic stress . . . might promote the initiation and progression of some types of cancer: Edna Maria Vissoci Reiche, Sandra Odebrecht Vargas Nunes, and Helena Kaminami Morimoto, "Stress, Depression, the Immune System, and Cancer." *The Lancet Oncology* 5, no. 10 (2004): 617–25; doi:10.1016/S1470-2045(04)01597-9.

91 victims of racism were more likely to have a limiting long-term illness: Kwame McKenzie, "Racism and Health." *BMJ (Clinical Research Ed.)* 326, no. 7380 (2003): 65–66; doi:10.1136/bmj.326.7380.65.

91 racism causes increased mortality rates: B. P. Kennedy et al., "(Dis)respect and Black Mortality." *Ethnicity & Disease* 7, no. 3 (1997): 207–14; http://europepmc .org/abstract/MED/9467703.

92 copycat suicides: M. S. Gould and D. Shaffer, "The Impact of Suicide in Television Movies. Evidence of Imitation." *New England Journal of Medicine* 315, no. 11 (1986): 690–94; doi:10.1056/NEJM198609113151107.

93 inhalation of toxic gases: N. Kreitman, "The Coal Gas Story. United Kingdom Suicide Rates, 1960–71." *British Journal of Preventive & Social Medicine* 30, no. 2 (1976): 86–93; doi:10.1136/jech.30.2.86.

93 link between overall state firearm ownership and firearm suicide: M. Miller, D. Azrael, and C. Barber, "Suicide Mortality in the United States: The Importance of Attending to Method in Understanding Population-level Disparities in the Burden of Suicide." *Annual Review of Public Health* 33 (2012): 393–408; doi:10.1146/ annurev-publhealth-031811-124636.

WEIGHT

103 increase in rates of obesity in the United States over the period of time from 1985 to 2010: CDC, "Obesity Trends Among U.S. Adults Between 1985 and 2010"; https://www.cdc.gov/obesity/downloads/obesity_trends_2010.pdf.

111 an increased suicide rate in the ten years after bariatric surgery: Hilary A. Tindle et al., "Risk of Suicide After Long-Term Follow-Up from Bariatric Surgery." *American Journal of Medicine* 123, no. 11 (2010): 1036–42; doi:10.1016/j.amjmed.2010.06.016.

BELIEF

120 the diagnosis of ADHD in childhood is greatly increased: Timothy J. Layton et al., "Attention Deficit–Hyperactivity Disorder and Month of School Enrollment." *New England Journal of Medicine* 379, no. 22 (2018): 2122–30; doi:10.1056/NEJMoa1806828.

121 had 128 categories and was 132 pages long: R. K. Blashfield, J. W. Keeley, E. H. Flanagan, and S. R. Miles, "The Cycle of Classification: DSM-I Through DSM-5." *Annual Review of Clinical Psychology* 10 (2014): 25–51; doi:10.1146/annurev-clinpsy-032813-153639.

122 Dunning and Kruger demonstrated: Justin Kruger and David Dunning, "Unskilled and Unaware of It: How Difficulties in Recognizing One's Own Incompetence Lead to Inflated Self-Assessments." *Journal of Personality and Social Psychology* 77, no. 6 (2000): 1121–34; doi:10.1037//0022-3514.77.6.1121.

124 In 2019, the CDC reported 1,282 cases of measles: Centers for Disease Control and Prevention, "Measles Cases and Outbreaks," last reviewed December 2, 2020; https://www.cdc.gov/measles/cases-outbreaks.html.

124 In Europe, the picture is even worse: World Health Organization, "Over 100,000 People Sick with Measles in 14 Months," May 9, 2019; http://www.euro.who.int/en/media-centre/sections/press-releases/2019/over-100-000-people-sick-with-measles-in-14-months-with-measles-cases-at-an-alarming-level-in-the-european-region,-who-scales-up-response.

125 48,000 were hospitalized, 1,000 developed encephalitis: Centers for Disease Control and Prevention, "Measles History," last reviewed November 5, 2020; https://www.cdc.gov/measles/about/history.html.

126 One study showed an increase in more educated people: J. A. Astin, "Why Patients Use Alternative Medicine: Results of a National Study." *JAMA* 279, no. 19 (1998): 1548–53; doi:10.1001/jama.279.19.1548.

127 Americans spend $30 billion a year on alternative health: Richard L. Nahin, Patricia M. Barnes, and Barbara J. Stussman, "Expenditures on Complementary Health Approaches: United States, 2012." *National Health Statistics Reports* 95 (2016): 1–11; https://www.researchgate.net/publication/304582545_Expenditures_on_Complementary_Health_Approaches_United_States_2012.

MEDICAL MYSTERIES

135 a report for the World Health Organization: World Health Organization, "Adherence to Long-Term Therapies: Evidence for Action," 2003; https://www.who.int/chp/knowledge/publications/adherence_full_report.pdf.

137 1 percent of all inpatient hospital admissions: A. J. Sutherland and G. M. Rodin, "Factitious Disorders in a General Hospital Setting: Clinical Features and a Review of the Literature." *Psychosomatics* 31 (1990): 392–99; doi:10.1016/S0033-3182(90)72133-0.

138 The term "Munchausen's syndrome" comes from the fictional character: Régis Olry and Duane E. Haines, "Chapter 7. Historical and Literary Roots of Münchhausen Syndromes: As Intriguing as the Syndromes Themselves," in S. Finger, F. Boller, and A. Stiles, eds., *Literature, Neurology, and Neuroscience: Neurological and Psychiatric Disorders* (Elsevier, 2013); http://www.sciencedirect.com/science/article/pii/B9780444633644000247.

MEANING

149 airline staff were concerned enough about the behavior of the terrorists: Mark G. Frank, Carl J. Maccario, and Venugopal Govindaraju, "Behavior and Security," in Paul Seidenstat and Francis X. Splane, eds., *Protecting Airline Passengers in the Age of Terrorism* (Praeger, 2009): 86–106.

151 As Andrew Malleson writes: Andrew Malleson, *Whiplash and Other Useful Illnesses* (McGill-Queen's University Press, 2005): 276.

154 I began to think of Viktor Frankl's: Viktor Frankl, *Man's Search for Meaning* (Simon & Schuster, 1985).

155 they have not got depression at all, but a life that lacks any higher goals: A.M. Santhouse, "The Person in the Patient." *BMJ* 337 (2008): a2262; doi: 10.1136/BMJ.A2262.

155 an article in *The New York Times* about Japanese labor laws: Hiroko Tabuchi, "Layoffs Taboo, Japan Workers Are Sent to the Boredom Room." *New York Times,* August 16, 2013.

ACCEPTANCE

163 women with eating disorders had a distorted view of their own bodies: Jonathan Guez et al., "Self-Figure Drawings in Women with Anorexia; Bulimia; Overweight; and Normal Weight: A Possible Tool for Assessment." *Arts in Psychotherapy* 37, no. 5 (2010): 400–406; doi:10.1016/j.aip.2010.09.001.

163 Genetic studies have examined differences: K. L. Klump et al., "Genetic and Environmental Influences on Anorexia Nervosa Syndromes in a Population-Based Twin Sample." *Psychological Medicine* 31, no. 4 (2001): 737–40; doi:10.1017/s0033291701003725.

164 **passed legislation that prohibited models:** Selina Sykes. "Six Countries Taking Steps to Tackle Super-skinny Models." *Euronews*, June 9, 2017; https://www.eu ronews.com/2017/09/06/counties-fighting-underweight-modelling.

164 **One of the most unusual studies:** A. E. Becker et al., "Eating Behaviors and Attitudes Following Prolonged Exposure to Television Among Ethnic Fijian Adolescent Girls." *British Journal of Psychiatry* 180 (2002): 509–14; doi:10.1192/bjp .180.6.509.

165 **anorexia has the highest mortality rate of any mental illness:** C. Harris and B. Barraclough, "Excess Mortality of Mental Disorder." *British Journal of Psychiatry* 173, no. 1 (1998): 11–53; doi:10.1192/bjp.173.1.11; Jon Arcelus et al., "Mortality Rates in Patients with Anorexia Nervosa and Other Eating Disorders. A Meta-Analysis of 36 Studies." *Archives of General Psychiatry* 68, no. 7 (2011): 724–31; doi:10.1001/archgenpsychiatry.2011.74.

169 **is predicted to be worth globally around $81 billion by 2024:** "Male Grooming Products Market: Global Industry Trends, Share, Size, Growth, Opportunity and Forecast 2019–2024," June 2019; https://www.researchandmarkets.com/reports /4775701/male-grooming-products-market-global-industry.

170 **newspaper feature that asked whether we will ever see "a cure for baldness":** Richard Godwin, "How Close Is a Cure for Baldness?," *The Guardian*, September 2, 2018; https://www.theguardian.com/fashion/2018/sep/02/hair-today-gone-tomorrow.

171 **homosexuality was defined as an illness right up until 1973:** J. Drescher, "Out of DSM: Depathologizing Homosexuality," *Behavioral Sciences* 5, no. 4 (2015): 565–75; doi:10.3390/bs5040565.

171 **Carl Rogers, an important, although now largely forgotten, figure of twentieth-century psychology:** Brian Thorne and Pete Sanders, *Carl Rogers*, 3rd ed. (SAGE Publications, 2013).

PAIN

174 **Aristotle, the Ancient Greek philosopher, maintained that the brain:** Edwin Clarke and Jerry Stannard, "Aristotle on the Anatomy of the Brain." *Journal of the History of Medicine and Allied Sciences* 18, no. 2 (1963): 130–48; doi:10.1093 /jhmas/XVIII.2.130.

175 **Descartes imagined as hollow tubes carrying "animal spirits" up to the brain:** Massieh Moayedi and Karen D. Davis, "Theories of Pain: From Specificity to Gate Control." *Journal of Neurophysiology* 109, no. 1 (2013): 5–12; doi:10.1152 /jn.00457.2012.

176 **In an often-cited paper from the 1960s:** R. Melzack and P. D. Wall, "Pain Mechanisms: A New Theory." *Science* 150 (1965): 71–979.

177 **chronic pain can be thought of as its own separate disease:** Irene Tracey and M. Catherine Bushnell, "How Neuroimaging Studies Have Challenged Us to

Rethink: Is Chronic Pain a Disease?" *Journal of Pain* 10, no. 11 (2009): 1113–20; doi:10.1016/j.jpain.2009.09.001.

180 **Zborowski selected ethnocultural groups:** Mark Zborowski, "Cultural Components in Responses to Pain." *Journal of Social Issues* 8, no. 4 (1952): 16–30; doi:10.1111/j.1540-4560.1952.tb01860.x.

181 **the Jewish volunteers knew the cause of the pain:** B. Berthold Wolff and Sarah Langley, "Cultural Factors and the Response to Pain: A Review." *American Anthropologist* 70, no. 3 (1968): 494–501; doi:10.1525/aa.1968.70.3.02a00030.

182 **which religious group could tolerate the greatest pain:** Wallace E. Lambert, Eva Libman, and Earnest G. Poser, "The Effect of Increased Salience of a Membership Group on Pain Tolerance." *Journal of Personality* 28 (1960): 350–57; doi:10.1111/j.1467-6494.1960.tb01624.x.

182 **a fascinating chapter included in a book about pain:** G. B. Rollman, "Ethnocultural Variations in the Experience of Pain," in T. Hadjistavropoulos and K. D. Craig, eds., *Pain: Psychological Perspectives* (Lawrence Erlbaum Associates, 2004): 155–78.

182 **Japanese patients are said to express pain:** G. B. Rollman, "Culture and Pain," in Shahé S. Kazarian and David R. Evans, eds., *Cultural Clinical Psychology: Theory, Research, and Practice* (Oxford University Press, 1998): 267–286.

182 **The English language often uses metaphor:** Elena Semino, "Descriptions of Pain, Metaphor, and Embodied Simulation." *Metaphor and Symbol* 25, no. 4 (2010): 205–26; doi:10.1080/10926488.2010.510926.

185 **individuals in a trial were asked to walk through exactly the same virtual reality library:** Daniel Freeman et al., "Can Virtual Reality Be Used to Investigate Persecutory Ideation?" *Journal of Nervous and Mental Disease* 191, no. 8 (2003): 509–14; doi:10.1097/01.nmd.0000082212.83842.fe.

185 **Depressed patients experience more physical symptoms:** G. E. Simon, M. VonKorff, M. Piccinelli, C. Fullerton, J. Ormel. "An International Study of the Relation Between Somatic Symptoms and Depression," *New England Journal of Medicine* 341, no. 18 (1999): 1329–35. doi:10.1056/NEJM199910283411801.

186 **classic novel about junior doctors:** Samuel Shem, *The House of God* (Black Swan, 1978).

186 **the 1958 cohort:** Gareth T. Jones, Chris Power, and Gary J. Macfarlane, "Adverse Events in Childhood and Chronic Widespread Pain in Adult Life: Results from the 1958 British Birth Cohort Study." *Pain* 143, no. 1–2 (2009): 92–96; doi:10.1016/j.pain.2009.02.003.

187 **One large U.S. study showed a relationship between adverse childhood experiences:** Vincent J. Felitti et al., "Relationship of Childhood Abuse and Household Dysfunction to Many of the Leading Causes of Death in Adults. The Adverse Childhood Experiences (ACE) Study." *American Journal of Preventive Medicine* 14, no. 4 (1998): 245–58; doi:10.1016/s0749-3797(98)00017-8.

WISHING FOR THE END

199 expanded to include patients with psychiatric disorders: Paul S. Appelbaum, "Physician-Assisted Death in Psychiatry." *World Psychiatry* 17, no. 2 (2018): 145–46; doi:10.1002/wps.20548.

199 3 percent of Belgian: Monica Verhofstadt, Lieve Thienpont, and Gjalt-Jorn Ygram Peters, "When Unbearable Suffering Incites Psychiatric Patients to Request Euthanasia: Qualitative Study." *British Journal of Psychiatry* 211, no. 4 (2017): 238–45; doi:10.1192/bjp.bp.117.199331.

199 Dutch assisted deaths: Agnes van der Heide, Johannes J. M. van Delden, and Bregje D. Onwuteaka-Philipsen, "End-of-Life Decisions in the Netherlands over 25 Years." *New England Journal of Medicine* 377, no. 5 (2017): 492–94; doi:10.1056/NEJMc1705630.

199 50 percent of Dutch psychiatric patients asking to die had a personality disorder: Scott Y. H. Kim, Raymond G. De Vries, and John R. Peteet, "Euthanasia and Assisted Suicide of Patients with Psychiatric Disorders in the Netherlands 2011 to 2014." *JAMA Psychiatry* 73, no. 4 (2016): 362–68; doi:10.1001/jamapsychiatry.2015.2887.

199 a figure similar to that in Belgium: Lieve Thienpont et al., "Euthanasia Requests, Procedures and Outcomes for 100 Belgian Patients Suffering from Psychiatric Disorders: A Retrospective, Descriptive Study." *BMJ Open* 5 (2015): e007454; doi:10.1136/bmjopen-2014-007454.

199 in 12 percent of such cases in the Netherlands, the three assessors: Samuel N. Doernberg, John R. Peteet, and Scott Y. H. Kim, "Capacity Evaluations of Psychiatric Patients Requesting Assisted Death in the Netherlands." *Psychosomatics* 57, no. 6 (2016): 556–65; doi:10.1016/j.psym.2016.06.005.

199 the general public are largely in favor of assisted dying: NatCen Social Research, "Moral Issues." *British Social Attitudes* 34 (2017); https://www.bsa.natcen.ac.uk/media/39147/bsa34_moral_issues_final.pdf.

199 Of those doctors working in palliative care or in elderly care: C. Seale, "Legalisation of Euthanasia or Physician-Assisted Suicide: Survey of Doctors' Attitudes." *Palliative Medicine* 23, no. 3 (2009): 205–12; doi:10.1177/0269216308102041.

THE PRICE OF A TROUBLED MIND

209 the King's Fund report: Chris Naylor et al., "Long-Term Conditions and Mental Health: The Cost of Co-Morbidities." The King's Fund and Centre for Mental Health, February 2012; https://www.kingsfund.org.uk/sites/default/files/field/field_publication_file/long-term-conditions-mental-health-cost-comorbidities-naylor-feb12.pdf.

209 In the United States, a study examining over 600,000 insurance claims: Charles A. Welch et al., "Depression and Costs of Health Care." *Psychosomatics* 50, no. 4 (2009): 392–401; doi:10.1176/appi.psy.50.4.392.

209 **A German study of over 300,000 patients:** Jan Wolff et al., "Hospital Costs Associated with Psychiatric Comorbidities: A Retrospective Study." *BMC Health Services Research* 18, no. 1 (2018): 67; doi:10.1186/s12913-018-2892-5.

209 **depression worsens the outcome after a stroke:** Ellen M. Whyte and Benoit H. Mulsant, "Post Stroke Depression: Epidemiology, Pathophysiology, and Biological Treatment." *Biological Psychiatry* 52, no. 3 (2002): 253–64; doi: 10.1016/s0006-3223(02)01424-5.

209 **the same is true of depression and heart disease:** Arup K. Dhar and David A. Barton, "Depression and the Link with Cardiovascular Disease." *Frontiers in Psychiatry* 7 (2016): 33; doi:10.3389/fpsyt.2016.00033.

210 **Patients with diseases of the airways:** A. I. Yang, T. A. Rolls, and D. L. Ward, "Anxiety and Depression—Important Psychological Comorbidities of COPD," *Journal of Thoracic Disease* 6, no. 11 (2014): 1615–31; doi:10.3978/j.issn.2072 -1439.2014.09.28.

210 **people with diabetes who develop depression:** Dominique L. Musselman et al., "Relationship of Depression to Diabetes Types 1 and 2: Epidemiology, Biology, and Treatment." *Biological Psychiatry* 54, no. 3 (2003): 317–29; doi:10.1016/s0006 -3223(03)00569-9.

211 **there is something about depression itself that seems to be toxic:** Lawson R. Wulsin, George E. Vaillant, and Victoria E. Wells, "A Systematic Review of the Mortality of Depression." *Psychosomatic Medicine* 61, no. 1 (1999): 6–17; doi: 10.1097/00006842-199901000-00003.

CAPACITY

219–20 **Psychiatry has always had an uneasy relationship with personality disorders . . . these labels are given to people who doctors just don't like:** G. Lewis and L. Appleby, "Personality Disorder: The Patients Psychiatrists Dislike." *British Journal of Psychiatry* 153 (1988): 44–49; doi:10.1192/bjp.153.1.44.

223 **at least 40 percent of patients admitted to a medical ward:** Vanessa Raymont et al., "Prevalence of Mental Incapacity in Medical Inpatients and Associated Risk Factors: Cross-Sectional Study." *Lancet* 364, no. 9443 (2004): 1421–27; doi:10.1016/ S0140-6736(04)17224-3.

227 **Dr. Tony Zigmond:** Tony Zigmond, *A Clinician's Brief Guide to the Mental Health Act* (RCPsych Publications, 2012).

FINAL DAYS

235 **the number one regret of the dying:** Bronnie Ware, "Regrets of the Dying," https://bronnieware.com/blog/regrets-of-the-dying.

236 **Chochinov explored the desire for death:** H. M. Chochinov et al., "Desire for Death in the Terminally Ill." *American Journal of Psychiatry* 152, no. 8 (1995): 1185–91; doi:10.1176/ajp.152.8.1185.

237 As Andrew Scull outlines: Andrew Scull, *Madness in Civilization: A Cultural History of Insanity, from the Bible to Freud, from the Madhouse to Modern Medicine* (Princeton University Press, 2015).

241 a 1979 study from Finland published in the *American Journal of Epidemiology*: K. A. Louhivuori and M. Hakama, "Risk of Suicide Among Cancer Patients." *American Journal of Epidemiology* 109, no. 1 (1979): 59–65; doi:10.1093/oxford journals.aje.a112659.

241 A more recent study in 2012 followed up on over 3.5 million people: Timothy V. Johnson et al., "Peak Window of Suicides Occurs Within the First Month of Diagnosis: Implications for Clinical Oncology." *Psycho-Oncology* 21, no. 4 (2012): 351–56; doi:10.1002/pon.1905.

241 about his treatment called Dignity Therapy: H. M. Chochinov et al., "Dignity Therapy: A Novel Psychotherapeutic Intervention for Patients Near the End of Life." *Journal of Clinical Oncology* 23, no. 24 (2005): 5520–25; doi:10.1200/JCO.2005.08.391.

242 undoubtedly helpful to their families, too: Susan McClement et al., "Dignity Therapy: Family Member Perspectives." *Journal of Palliative Medicine* 10, no. 5 (2007): 1076–82; doi:10.1089/jpm.2007.0002.

242 a different study in the *British Medical Journal*: Courtney Davis et al., "Availability of Evidence of Benefits on Overall Survival and Quality of Life of Cancer Drugs Approved by European Medicines Agency: Retrospective Cohort Study of Drug Approvals 2009–13." *BMJ* 359 (2017): j4530; doi:10.1136/bmj.j4530.

COVID

245 a term borrowed from the military, that of "moral injury": Brett T. Litz et al., "Moral Injury and Moral Repair in War Veterans: A Preliminary Model and Intervention Strategy." *Clinical Psychology Review* 29, no. 8 (2009): 695–706; doi:10.1016/j.cpr.2009.07.003.

245 "We did all that we could": N. Greenberg, M. Docherty, S. Gnanapragasam, and S. Wessely, "Managing Mental Health Challenges Faced by Healthcare Workers During Covid-19 Pandemic," *BMJ* 368 (2020); doi:10.1136/bmj.m1211.

246 The paper examined the suicide rates after the terrorist attacks: E. Salib, "Effect of 11 September 2001 on Suicide and Homicide in England and Wales." *British Journal of Psychiatry* 183, no. 3 (2003): 207–12; doi:10.1192/bjp.183.3.207.

246 the theories of Émile Durkheim: Émile Durkheim, *Suicide: A Study in Sociology* (Routledge & Kegan Paul, 1952 [1897]).

249 the well-known Whitehall study: H. Bosma et al., "Low Job Control and Risk of Coronary Heart Disease in Whitehall II (Prospective Cohort) Study." *BMJ* 314, no. 7080 (1997): 558–65; doi:10.1136/bmj.314.7080.558.

EPILOGUE

259 **a doctor will typically interrupt after eleven seconds:** Naykky Singh Ospina et al., "Eliciting the Patient's Agenda—Secondary Analysis of Recorded Clinical Encounters." *Journal of General Internal Medicine* 34, no. 1 (2019): 36–40; doi:10.1007/s11606-018-4540-5.

263 **later published in his excellent blog:** Jonathan Glass, "The Heart Sink Doctor." *The BMJ Opinion,* October 23, 2019; https://blogs.bmj.com/bmj/2019/10/23/jonathan-glass-the-heart-sink-doctor.

266 **In the UK we spend £8 to £13 billion extra per annum:** Chris Naylor et al., "Long-Term Conditions and Mental Health: The Cost of Co-Morbidities." The King's Fund and Centre for Mental Health, February 2012; https://www.kingsfund.org.uk/sites/default/files/field/field_publication_file/long-term-conditions-mental-health-cost-comorbidities-naylor-feb12.pdf.

266 **the costs of medically unexplained symptoms are $256 billion per annum:** Arthur J. Barsky, E. John Orav, and David W. Bates, "Somatization Increases Medical Utilization and Costs Independent of Psychiatric and Medical Comorbidity." *Archives of General Psychiatry* 62, no. 8 (2005): 903–10; doi:10.1001/archpsyc.62.8.903.

INDEX